Introductory Neurology

Introductory Neurology

James G. McLeod
AO, MB BS, BSc(Med), DPhil(Oxon),
FRCP, FRACP, FAA, FTS
*Bushell Professor of Neurology and
Bosch Professor of Medicine,
University of Sydney;
Head, Department of Neurology,
Royal Prince Alfred Hospital, Sydney*

James W. Lance
CBE, MD, FRCP, FRACP, FAA
*Chairman, Department of Neurology,
Prince Henry and Prince of Wales
Hospitals; Professor of Neurology,
University of New South Wales, Sydney*

SECOND EDITION

Blackwell Scientific Publications
MELBOURNE OXFORD LONDON
EDINBURGH BOSTON

© 1983, 1989 by
Blackwell Scientific Publications
Editorial Offices:
107 Barry Street, Carlton
   Victoria 3053 Australia
Osney Mead, Oxford OX2 0EL
   (*Orders:* Tel. 0865 240201)
8 John Street, London WC1N 2ES
23 Ainslie Place, Edinburgh EH3 6AJ
3 Cambridge Center, Suite 208,
   Cambridge, Massachusetts 02142, USA

First published 1983
Reprinted with corrections 1986
Second edition published 1989

Typeset in Baskerville by
Abb-typesetting Pty Ltd, Melbourne
Printed in Singapore by
Kin Keong Printing Co. Pte. Ltd.

DISTRIBUTORS
USA
   Year Book Medical Publishers
   200 North LaSalle Street
   Chicago, Illinois 60601
   (*Orders:* Tel. 312 726-9733)

Canada
   The C.V. Mosby Company
   5420 Finch Avenue East
   Scarborough, Ontario
   (*Orders:* Tel. 416 298-1588)

Australia
   Blackwell Scientific
   Publications (Australia) Pty Ltd
   107 Barry Street,
   Carlton, Victoria 3053
   (*Orders:* Tel. 03 347 0300)

Cataloguing in Publication Data

Introductory neurology.

   2nd ed.
   Includes bibliographies and index.
   ISBN 0 86793 017 9.

   1. Neurology. I. McLeod, James G.
   (James Graham). II. Lance, James W.
   (James Waldo), 1926–

616.8

The cover illustration is a stylized version of the spinal cord and roots. (After Shadé, 1966, *The Peripheral Nervous System.* Elsevier Publishing Company, Amsterdam.)

Contents

Preface to the Second Edition

The first edition has been completely revised and, in order to make the coverage of neurological conditions more comprehensive, new chapters on the autonomic nervous system, dementia, degenerative diseases, and treatment of neurological disorders have been added. There are 33 new figures, and we are grateful to Mr Robert Haynes of the Department of Audiovisual Services, Royal Prince Alfred Hospital for the new line drawings.

J.G. McLeod and J.W. Lance

Preface to the First Edition

The present book is designed to help the undergraduate medical student relate already acquired knowledge of the basic neurological sciences to the examination of the patient and to diseases of the nervous system. There has been no attempt to discuss in detail all the conditions seen by a neurologist and their treatment since there are many excellent comprehensive textbooks readily available which can and should be consulted. The physiological mechanisms of symptoms and signs are discussed only briefly since the subject has been considered by the authors in another book, *A Physiological Approach to Clinical Neurology* (3rd edn, 1981, Butterworths, London). We are greatly indebted to our colleagues, particularly to Drs R.A. Ouvrier and P.G. Procopis, who have contributed so much by their discussions and in their lectures: to J. Eichorn, L. Hansen and F. Rubiu for the line drawings; and to D. Jones for typing the manuscript.

J.G. McLeod and J.W. Lance

1 History Taking

Most patients present to their doctors with a problem, with some observations about themselves or symptoms that they consider abnormal or indicative of ill-health. The first and most important measure in helping patients to solve their problems is to take a detailed unhurried history of the development of symptoms and their evolution, and then to assess this with a knowledge of the patient's family and personal background. In some neurological disorders, it may be possible to reach a firm diagnosis on the history alone. The acquisition of the clinical skills of history taking and physical examination may eliminate the need for further investigations or at least limit these to the minimum necessary to achieve a final diagnosis. The process of history taking involves a number of steps. The precise sequence in which these steps are taken may vary from one medical school to another, from one doctor to another, or even for the same doctor dealing with different problems. The important point is that the thought process should be logical and should lead to a conclusion. Each aspect of the history should be stated as precisely as possible and not glossed over in general terms.

Before the history is taken, the details of the patient's name, address, date of birth, occupation and other necessary data are recorded. After a general enquiry about the purpose of the consultation, notes may be taken about the patient's personal background, family history and past health before going into detail about the problems which chiefly concern him or her. Alternatively, the problem may be analysed carefully as the 'history of the present illness' and then the past, family and personal histories recorded afterwards. The latter approach will be taken to illustrate the case-history of a hypothetical patient, a woman aged 40 years, with a neurological problem.

Presenting symptoms and signs (and their duration)

Weakness of both legs, 2 years; numbness of both legs, 1 year; urgency of micturition, 6 months.

History of the present illness

This section can be presented in note form or as a narrative, recorded as it unfolds from the patient's own account, sharpened a little here and there by an occasional direct question from the clinician to keep the history within the bounds of relevance and to prevent it from degenerating into a list of doctors consulted, investigations ordered and opinions proffered by neighbours and casual acquaintances.

The nature of the symptoms elicited makes the clinician think in terms of localization of the disorder in the nervous system, whether it originates in cerebral hemispheres, brainstem, cerebellum, spinal cord, spinal roots, peripheral nerve or muscle, or whether it may be the product of a troubled mind.

The pattern of evolution of symptoms, whether steadily progressive, fluctuating in intensity or remitting for long periods, guides the clinician in assessing the likely pathological cause of the lesion or lesions. In the example given above, the restriction of motor and sensory symptoms to the lower limbs makes one think of a spinal cord lesion and the association with urgency of micturition (disinhibition of bladder reflexes) places the lesion above the conus medullaris, i.e. in the thoracic spinal cord. If the condition is steadily progressive, compression of the spinal cord or a lesion within the spinal cord is likely and warrants immediate investigation. If the condition has fluctuated or remitted one has to entertain the diagnosis of multiple sclerosis. It is important to gauge from the history the *upper limit* of any lesion, if possible. If the patient cited above has also noticed paraesthesiae in the little fingers of both hands, the lesion must be at the level of the eighth cervical segment or above (Fig. 1.1).

Any associated features, precipitating or relieving factors for the symptoms may give a clue as to their nature. This is particularly important in taking a history of any pain, including headache, which should include the following information.

Pain history

Length of history: when did the pain first start?
Site: precise part of head, neck, back or other area involved.
Radiation: the distribution of any radicular pain is important for localization (Figs 1.1, 1.2), e.g. low back pain may radiate to the medial malleolus (L4 segment), the outer malleolus (L5 segment), and the back of the heel (S1 segment). Pain is referred to a sclerotome.
Quality of pain: e.g. stabbing (tic douloureux, lightning pains); throbbing, pulsatile (indicating a vascular component); burning (indicating small sensory fibre involvement); constant, tight, colicky, etc.

Fig. 1.1 Dermatomes and sclerotomes in the upper limb. If one nerve root only is damaged, sensory loss is usually restricted to the dotted areas shown on the left. Paraesthesiae are generally referred to the dermatome and pain to the sclerotome. (From Lance and McLeod, 1981, with permission of Butterworths, London.)

Fig. 1.2 Dermatomes and sclerotomes of the lower limbs. (From Lance and McLeod, 1981, with permission of Butterworths, London.)

Frequency of pain: continuous or intermittent. How many times felt in each day or week?

Duration of pain: seconds, minutes, hours.

Time of onset: any habitual pattern? Awakening from sleep? At the end of the day?

Mode of onset: sudden, slowly progressive or preceded by other symptoms, e.g. visual disturbance at the onset of migraine headache.

Associated features: nausea, vomiting, dyspnoea, palpitations or other symptoms.

Precipitating factors: movement of head, neck or back. Coughing, sneezing, straining.

Relieving factors: certain postures, pressure over the affected part, bedrest, heat or cold, various medications and their effects.

With any syndrome, the symptoms *first* noticed at the onset and the circumstances in which they appeared are of primary importance in determining the site of origin and possible cause.

Specific interrogation

After the history of the present illness has been clarified as far as possible, the clinician runs through a check list of neurological symptoms to ensure that nothing of relevance has been overlooked, starting at the top of the nervous system and working downwards, asking about the following symptoms:

Intellectual changes, confusion or loss of memory.

Headaches, fits or faints, drowsiness.

Speech disturbance — dysphasia (is the patient right or left handed?); dysarthria; dysphonia.

Sense of smell (cranial nerve 1).

Visual acuity (cranial nerve 2) — impairment or hallucinations of vision; limited to one eye, one half field or bilateral?; details and duration.

Double vision (cranial nerves 3, 4, 6).

Facial paraesthesiae or numbness (cranial nerve 5).

Facial weakness (cranial nerve 7).

If facial palsy is apparent from the history, was it accompanied by hyperacusis or impairment of taste on the affected side?

Hearing, tinnitus and vertigo (cranial nerve 8).

Swallowing, coughing and quality of speech (cranial nerves 9, 10, 12 and central portion of 11).

Weakness
  unilateral
    hemiparesis: cerebral or brainstem origin
    monoparesis: cerebral, spinal cord or roots

bilateral
> quadriparesis: cervical cord or above
> paraparesis: thoracic cord, conus or cauda equina

proximal: myopathy
distal: peripheral neuropathy
fatiguability: myasthenia gravis

Paraesthesiae or numbness — distribution of the same significance as weakness, with the additional information that (a) numbness of half of the face and opposite side of the body indicates a brainstem lesion; (b) burning sensations down one side of the body with weakness of the other side suggests a unilateral spinal cord lesion (Brown-Séquard syndrome); (c) paraesthesiae from a spinal root disturbance are referred to a *dermatome* (Figs 1.1, 1.2).

Specific symptoms (common in multiple sclerosis) to be asked about are: (a) tingling down the back on flexing the neck (Lhermitte's sign, electric shock sign) indicating a lower cervical lesion; (b) band-like sensations around the trunk or pelvis; (c) tight wrapping sensations around the legs. The last two symptoms are from dorsal root entry zones or dorsal columns.

Sphincter disturbance — urgency of, or difficulty in initiating micturition or defaecation; incontinence.

Impotence or failure of ejaculation.

Difficulty with coordination, balance or gait.

Other systems

Since the nervous system does not exist in isolation, the usual questions must be asked about other systems. Those of most relevance to neurological disorders are listed below.

Systemic disturbances, such as connective tissue diseases, malignancy or infections — loss of weight; fever, sweating; aches in muscles or joints.

Respiratory disease (such as carcinoma of the lung, tuberculosis, sarcoid, bronchiectasis) which may be related to neurological symptoms — tightness or pain in the chest; dyspnoea; haemoptysis.

Cardiovascular symptoms, often associated with cerebral vascular disease — palpitations (cardiac dysrhythmias); angina pectoris; intermittent claudication.

Endocrine disorders, drawing attention to the hypothalamus and area around the pituitary fossa — polyuria, polydipsia; symptoms of thyroid or pituitary dysfunction; unexplained weight change; loss of body hair; amenorrhoea, loss of libido, testicular atrophy.

Past history

One of the arts of history taking is to know what of the past history is relevant to the present illness or, indeed, whether it may actually form part of the present illness. If, for example, the patient whose presenting symptoms and signs were given at the beginning of this chapter eventually disclosed that she had suffered loss of vision in the right eye for a period of 3 weeks at the age of 27 years and a tight, band-like sensation around the trunk for 2 months at the age of 35 years, these previous episodes could well be listed at the beginning of the history and would draw attention to the multifocal nature of symptoms experienced by the patient, e.g. transient loss of vision aged 27, band-like sensation around the trunk aged 35, progressive weakness of the legs for the past 2 years.

In the case of epilepsy, mental retardation, or any illness that could have been present at the time of birth or may have been initiated by the birth process, the course of pregnancy and labour and birth-weight should be noted. Was the baby given immediately to the mother or was resuscitation, intensive care or a humidicrib required? Milestones of development, the time of sitting, standing, walking and talking, and progress at school, become relevant. Did the child suffer convulsions, with or without a fever? Some 10% of children with febrile convulsions have fits in later life. Head injury, meningitis or encephalitis are obviously of potential relevance to the onset of epilepsy.

A history of headaches, motion sickness, abdominal pain or episodes of vomiting ('bilious attacks') in childhood may augur the development of migraine in adult life.

Recurrent headaches with neck stiffness in the past (perhaps diagnosed as meningo-encephalitis) may suggest repeated bleeding from a cerebral angioma.

A history of diabetes, hypertension, tuberculosis, immune disorders or other serious illness should be recorded, as should any operation, even seemingly minor procedures such as the removal of a 'mole' from the skin.

Family history

Many neurological disorders like Huntington's chorea, the heredo-familial ataxias, Charcot-Marie-Tooth disease, muscular dystrophies and some forms of epilepsy are clearly of genetic origin. Other conditions such as migraine and cerebral vascular diseases tend to 'run in families' although no pattern of inheritance has been determined.

Personal and social background

The personality of the patient, his or her relationship with peer groups, spouse, children, and attitude to occupation may play an important part in the genesis of symptoms considered to be neurological, because of the constant interaction of mind and body. On the other hand, the development of neurological illness may have a profound impact on the patient's ability to work, to maintain satisfactory relationships with family and friends, and to derive benefit and enjoyment from life. One must therefore obtain as accurate a picture as possible of the type of life that a patient is leading and hopes to lead in the future to aid in diagnosis and then to help in counselling once the diagnosis is reached. The financial state of the family must also be assessed to see whether some form of financial assistance through sickness benefits or pensions is required. The emotional state of the patient must be carefully assessed as minor degrees of depression are very common and often relevant.

The nature of the patient's occupation and the details of his or her work must be noted because of the possible relevance to the neurological problem and in case of any Workers' Compensation or other legal action.

Standard questions about the amount of alcohol consumed, smoking habits, exposure to toxins and consumption of drugs are also of importance. The patient should be asked to list all medications currently being consumed or that have been used in the past since they may be relevant to present symptoms and certainly must be known to the clinician before any pharmaceutical agent is prescribed. Tactful enquiry about sexual preference has become increasingly important as the neurological manifestations of acquired immune-deficiency syndrome (AIDS) are more often encountered.

Guide to diagnosis from the history

The concept of taking such a complete medical history may seem daunting to those who are just starting their clinical training. With greater experience the process becomes easier and quicker, and is spiced with interest or even excitement as the clues present themselves to the receptive mind of the clinician. The phlegmatic recording of the history without any attempt being made by the clinician to correlate the facts as they appear, to make deductions and to form a provisional diagnosis during the process, can be a fruitless exercise. The pieces of the puzzle must be fitted into place while the story is evolving so that any missing fragments can be sought later.

The aim of history taking is to establish as far as possible whether the illness is likely to be of organic or psychological origin. If it is organic, what part or parts of the nervous system may be implicated? What is the pattern of the illness over a period of time? What are the precipitating and relieving factors? What is the possible pathology?

Particular attention should be paid to the following points.

Localization

Do the symptoms arise in one site or multiple sites? Can they be explained on the basis of impairment of a particular system (e.g. posterior columns, spinocerebellar pathways, corticospinal tracts) or a particular vascular territory (internal carotid and its branches, vertebrobasilar system, anterior spinal artery)?

Examples of symptoms arising from various sites are:

Cortex   Focal (partial) epileptic seizures. Localizing cerebral symptoms (see Chapter 12). Hemianopic or quadrantanopic field defects (see Chapter 9).

Thalamus   Contralateral dysaesthesiae (unpleasant burning pain) or sensory loss.

Basal ganglia   Parkinson's disease, involuntary movements (see Chapter 11).

Internal capsule   Contralateral hemiplegia (and sometimes limb ataxia) and sensory loss.

Midbrain   Tectum (superior colliculi): failure of upward deviation of the eyes (Parinaud's syndrome). Tegmentum: third nerve palsy. Contralateral 'wing-beating' (red nucleus) tremor. Contralateral hemiparesis.

Pons and medulla   Ipsilateral facial numbness (and often contralateral numbness of the body). Paresis of sixth, seventh, ninth, tenth or twelfth cranial nerves. Dysarthria and dysphagia from involvement of cranial nerves 9–12 is called 'bulbar palsy'. If impairment of speech and swallowing is caused by involvement of corticobulbar pathways rostral to lower cranial nerve nuclei, the condition is called 'pseudobulbar palsy'. Vertigo, tinnitus, deafness (eighth cranial nerve). Ipsilateral

Horner's syndrome (sympathetic pathway). Contralateral hemiparesis. Ipsilateral cerebellar signs. Sometimes a lesion in the upper pons may compromise corticopontocerebellar fibres so that limb ataxia is on the same side as the hemiparesis ('ataxic hemiparesis').

Cerebellum Midline: vertigo; ataxia of gait. Hemispheres: ipsilateral incoordination (see Chapter 10).

Spinal cord (see Chapter 8) Bilateral: motor and sensory loss below the level of the lesion. Sparing of posterior columns suggests anterior cord compression or anterior spinal artery involvement. Urgency of micturition. Unilateral: ipsilateral paresis and loss of joint position sense with contralateral loss of pinprick and temperature sensation (Brown-Séquard syndrome). The horizontal level is estimated from any accompanying lower motor neurone lesion, sensory impairment or reflex loss at the segment or segments involved and by the upper limit of the upper motor neurone and sensory tract involvement.

Roots Weakness, wasting, pain, paraesthesiae, or sensory, motor and reflex loss in the distribution of a particular root or roots as described above.

Peripheral nerves (see Chapter 5) Sensory and motor symptoms in the distribution of a particular nerve (mononeuritis), several nerves (mononeuritis multiplex) or all peripheral nerves symmetrically (peripheral neuropathy).

Neuromuscular junction (see Chapter 6) A purely motor syndrome with fatiguability (myasthenia). Muscles commonly involved are: extraocular muscles (ptosis, diplopia, without pupillary changes); bulbar muscles; proximal limb muscles.

Muscle (see Chapter 6) A purely motor syndrome with proximal wasting and weakness.

Mode of onset

Note the precise sequence of events at the onset of the illness. The initial story given might be one of loss of consciousness. 'I just blacked out, went out like a light'. 'Yes, but what were you doing at the time? Did you notice anything just before you became unconscious?'

Repeating this question in different form a number of times (because patients often think that minor sensations are of no significance and not worth reporting) often helps to diagnose the cause of the episode. Sample replies might include:

'Well, I just turned my head to one side, then my eyes went dim and I felt giddy' (vertebrobasilar insufficiency).

'My heart started racing and I felt faint' (cardiac dysrhythmia causing syncope).

'I just got out of bed to pass urine and woke up on the floor of the bathroom' (micturition syncope).

'My chest was tight and I couldn't get enough air into my lungs' (anxiety hyperventilation).

'I suddenly felt very frightened, as though it had all happened before' (temporal lobe epilepsy).

The principle is to look for the minor symptoms that lead to the major event, for they and they alone may hold the key to the diagnostic doorway.

The evolution (temporal pattern) of the illness

Have the symptoms reached their maximum and then progressively subsided?
For example:
    headache — viral meningo-encephalitis.
    vertigo, tinnitus — acute labyrinthitis.
    weakness — upper motor neurone: acute stroke;
                 — lower motor neurone: Guillain-Barré disease (acute polyneuritis).
Have the symptoms relapsed and remitted?
For example:
    headache — migraine.
    vertigo, tinnitus — Menière's syndrome.
    weakness — upper motor neurone: multiple sclerosis;
                 — lower motor neurone: relapsing polyneuritis.
Have the symptoms progressively become worse?
For example:
    headache — cerebral tumour or other space-occupying lesion.
    vertigo, tinnitus — acoustic neuroma or brainstem glioma.
    weakness — upper motor neurone and lower motor neurone: motor neurone disease (amyotrophic lateral sclerosis).

The temporal pattern thus gives some idea of the nature of the pathological process.

Conclusion

The history enables an hypothesis to be formed about the site of origin and cause of the patient's symptoms. The physical examination then tests aspects of this hypothesis. After that, further elucidation of the problem may depend on special investigations. Bear in mind that physical examination and diagnostic tests may not help. *Diagnosis often depends entirely on the history.*

2 Neurological Examination

General

Appearance and behaviour of the patient

During history taking, the emotional state and general intellectual competence of the patient will have become apparent, as well as any abnormal facial appearance, posture or involuntary movements.

Gait and stance

If the patient is able to walk, one observes body posture, swinging of the arms, and movements of the legs and feet, looking for asymmetry or any deviation from normal in the pace, fluidity of movement and maintenance of balance. Balance can be tested more stringently by asking the patient to walk *heel-to-toe*. The patient is then asked to stand with the feet together, then to close the eyes. If the patient is unable to maintain the upright posture with the eyes closed (Romberg's sign), proprioceptive information from the lower limbs is deficient.

The patient may be asked to hold the examiner's hands and to stand on the heels, elevating the feet, so that a minor degree of foot-drop can be observed.

Mental state

Level of consciousness

If the patient is stuporose, the level of consciousness may be assessed by responsiveness to voice, touch or painful stimuli. The examination of the unconscious or uncooperative patient is discussed in Chapter 13.

Orientation in time and place

Does the patient know the day, month and year, his or her usual address and the place where he or she is at the moment of examination?

General intellectual function

If patients are partly demented or confused, the degree of mental impairment can be gauged superficially by assessing spontaneous speech, the answers to simple questions about current affairs, the explanation of simple phrases, jokes or proverbs. An intellectually impaired patient may give a literal rather than a figurative interpretation — so-called 'concrete thought'. Evidence of serious emotional or thought disorder requires psychiatric consultation and evidence of dementia should be documented by formal psychometric testing.

Memory

If patients have recently suffered a head injury they should be asked for their last recollection before impact to assess the duration of *retrograde amnesia*, and their first memory after the accident to assess the duration of *post-traumatic amnesia*. If recent memory is defective, the patient may recite imaginary events to fill in the gaps ('confabulation', a feature of Korsakoff's psychosis). A commonly used test for registration and short-term retention of memory is to ask the patient to remember a name and address for 5 min while the examination continues. Digit span (normally seven numbers forward and five backwards) and the serial sevens test are other commonly used tests of mental function.

Speech and handedness

If speech is entirely normal, this should be stated and preference for using the right or left hand noted, since language is a function of the dominant hemisphere (the left hemisphere in over 50% of left-handers as well as in 96% of right-handers).

Speech defects should be described as: (a) Dysphasia — difficulty in understanding the spoken word or expressing thoughts in words, discussed further in Chapter 12. (b) Dysarthria — faulty articulation although word comprehension and selection are normal. (c) Dysphonia — impaired timbre of the voice from disorders of the vocal cords.

Localization of cortical dysfunction

If there is no perceptual or communication disorder this section may be omitted.

Disordered perception

Spoken word (sensory dysphasia: Wernicke area).
Written word (dyslexia: dominant parieto-occipital area).

Tactile recognition (agnosia: parietal lobe).
Visual or tactile inattention (unilateral neglect of bilaterally presented stimuli: parietal lobe).
Spatial relation to environment (losing way in familiar surroundings: non-dominant parietal lobe).

Disordered expression

Inability to select words and name objects (dysphasia: Broca and Wernicke areas); inability to write (dysgraphia: dominant parietal lobe); inability to calculate (acalculia: dominant parietal lobe); inability to distinguish right from left (right–left disorientation: dominant parietal lobe); inability to perform routine tasks (apraxia: dominant parietal or frontal lobes); inability to draw, construct diagrams (constructional apraxia: either parietal lobe); inability to dress oneself (non-dominant parietal lobe).

Skull

The size and shape of the skull are observed and the circumference measured if microcephaly or hydrocephalus are suspected (see Figs 2.1 and 2.2 for normal values). The skull may be palpated, with attention to the fontanelles in young children. When relevant (suspected angioma or vascular tumour), the examiner listens for a bruit over the orbits, temples and mastoid processes. For auscultation over the orbits, the patient is asked to close both eyes while the bell of the stethoscope is placed over one eye. The patient is then asked to open the other eye. This minimizes artefactual sounds from eyelid tremor.

Spine

The spine is examined for evidence of deformities, such as kyphosis, scoliosis or lordosis. The area of the spine appropriate to the symptoms is particularly inspected for any abnormality such as a tuft of hair in the lumbosacral region which may indicate an underlying spina bifida or other congenital anomaly. The cervical, thoracic or lumbar spine is then moved actively and passively through the full range to determine limitation of movement. Tenderness may be sought by pressure between the spinous processes and lateral to them (over the zygapophysial joints). Sometimes a smart blow over the suspected area of the spine may reproduce root pains but this test must be employed with discretion.

Resistance to flexing the neck (neck rigidity) is found with meningeal irritation (subarachnoid haemorrhage, meningitis) as well as with local

Fig. 2.1 Head circumference in girls. (From Nellhaus, 1968, *Pediatrics* **41**, 106, with permission of the author and publisher, copyright American Academy of Pediatrics, 1968.)

Fig. 2.2 Head circumference in boys. (From Nellhaus, 1968, *Pediatrics* **41**, 106, with permission of the author and publisher, copyright American Academy of Pediatrics, 1968.)

lesions. Another sign of meningeal irritation is inability to extend the leg at the knee joint when the lower limb is flexed at the hip (Kernig's sign).

In lumbosacral root irritation, *straight leg raising* (the extended lower limb being passively flexed at the hip joint by the examiner) is limited by pain on the affected side.

The examiner listens for a bruit over the carotid artery in patients with cerebral vascular insufficiency, and over the spine if an angioma is suspected.

Cranial nerves (see also Chapter 9)

Cranial nerve I (olfactory nerve)

It is important to test the sense of smell in patients with dementia (olfactory groove meningioma), ocular palsies (sphenoid wing meningioma) and after head injury (the olfactory nerve is often damaged by shearing strain at the moment of impact).

Cranial nerve II (optic nerve)

(a) Visual acuity, right and left, should be recorded at 6 m from a Snellen's chart, with the patient wearing glasses if necessary [e.g. VAR 6/6 VAL 6/9 (corrected)] — in the USA, normal vision is recorded (in feet) as 20/20.

(b) Ophthalmoscopic examination of the fundi. The key point in the examination of the fundi is for the patient to be able to fix on an external object with one eye while the other eye is being examined. This means that the examiner's head must remain vertical so as not to obscure the vision of the patient's fixating eye.

Note especially the optic disc — its colour (? pallor of the temporal half or the whole disc), the optic cup (enlarged in glaucoma, diminished in papilloedema), pulsation of the veins where they pass over the rim of the optic cup (absent in papilloedema) and the circumference of the disc (the disc is swollen and margins are blurred in papilloedema).

The state of the vessels in the periphery (arterio-venous nipping, haemorrhages, micro-aneurysms) is also noted and the surface of the retina scanned for abnormalities (exudates, choroiditis or retinitis pigmentosa).

(c) Visual fields. The patient is first confronted by the examiner, meeting his gaze, while the binocular fields are tested with the examiner's arms outstretched, moving the index finger on the right then the left hand, then both together in the outer quadrants of the fields of vision. In this way a complete homonymous hemianopia or visual inattention to one side can be detected.

Each eye is then tested individually with the other eye covered, the examiner bringing a finger, or preferably a white- or red-headed pin, from the periphery toward the centre of each quadrant. The blind spot should be defined and compared in size with that of the examiner. If a field defect is suspected it is advisable to advance the pin at right angles to the presumed junction between abnormal and normal parts of the visual field so that a scotoma, hemianopia or quadrantanopia can be clearly defined. Colour vision should also be tested with Ishihara test charts, particularly if optic neuritis past or present is suspected.

(d) Pupillary response to light, described below.

Cranial nerves III (oculomotor), IV (trochlear) and VI (abducens) and the ocular sympathetic nerve

(a) Orbit. Prominence of the eye (proptosis, exophthalmos) is noted.

(b) Ptosis. A partial ptosis may be congenital, myopathic, myasthenic or part of a Horner's syndrome (in which case the ipsilateral pupil will be small, and sweating may be impaired over the same side of the forehead). A complete ptosis is usually part of a third nerve palsy, in which case the pupil is usually dilated.

(c) Pupils. The size, shape and symmetry of the pupils are noted.

Pupillary responses (i) Accommodation. Normal pupils constrict as the eyes converge ('near response'). (ii) Light reflex. The normal pupil contracts briskly in the eye to which the light is directed (direct response) and also in the opposite eye (consensual response).

Afferent limb — optic nerve.

Efferent limb — Edinger-Westphal nucleus and third cranial nerve.

Assuming the third nerve is intact bilaterally, the optic nerve contribution to the reflex may be assessed by swinging a torch from one eye to the other. If there is impaired conduction in one optic nerve, the direct response to light in that eye will be insufficient to prevent dilatation of the pupil on that side as it recovers from the consensual constriction induced by shining the light in the sound eye. The effect will thus be pupillary constriction while the light is shone in the sound eye and pupillary dilatation when the light is swung to the eye on the affected side ('swinging torch sign' or Marcus Gunn sign).

(d) Ocular movements. Ocular movements are tested in the horizontal plane by asking the patient to look laterally to right and left (saccadic movements) and then to follow the examiner's finger to right and left (pursuit movements), maintaining the lateral position long enough to observe whether nystagmus develops. Vertical eye movements are tested with eyes looking to right and left as well as straight ahead in order to test the actions of the individual muscles. The patient should be asked if he sees a double image in any of the positions of gaze, and if so the paretic muscle should be identified (see p. 123). If nystagmus is present it should be further analysed (see p. 131).

Cranial nerve V (trigeminal nerve)

Motor

The patient is asked to open the jaw to ensure that it opens in the midline and does not deviate to one side (the jaw deviates to the side of a lower motor neurone lesion because of unequal action of the pterygoid muscles). The power of jaw closure is then tested and the masseter and temporalis muscles palpated. The pterygoid muscles may be tested separately by asking the patient to thrust the jaw sideways.

Sensory

Each of the three divisions of the trigeminal nerve is then tested by touch and pinprick with particular attention being paid to the anatomical distribution of sensory loss and to whether or not there is dissociation of painful and tactile sensation. Sensation on both sides of the face should be compared. Bear in mind that the territory of the second division extends only half-way between the nose and the angle of the mandible (Fig. 9.20). If a subtle lesion is suspected an added refinement is to test for two-point discrimination (the points being separated by 2 mm) on the lip of one side then the other.

Reflexes

(a) The corneal reflex is tested by applying a wisp of cotton wool to the lateral aspect of the cornea (not the conjunctiva); the stimulus induces a blink response. The examiner's hand rests on the patient's cheek so that the stimulus can be applied gently to the cornea, using the fingers with delicacy, and not by a frontal assault which induces a startle response.

Afferent pathway — trigeminal nerve, first division (part of the cornea is sometimes supplied by the second division).

Efferent pathway — facial nerve.

(b) The jaw jerk. A tap on the relaxed, partly open jaw with a percussion hammer evokes a barely perceptible contraction of the jaw-closing muscles in most normal subjects. An exaggerated jaw jerk is an important sign of a bilateral upper motor neurone lesion involving corticobulbar pathways.

Afferent pathway
Efferent pathway
} third division of trigeminal nerve.

(c) Glabella tap sign. Repeatedly tapping the mid-forehead at a rate of about 1/s induces a bilateral blink response, which is rapidly suppressed in most normal subjects. A continued blink response to each tap is often observed in Parkinson's disease. The mechanism is obscure.

Cranial nerve VII (facial nerve)

Motor

The face should be inspected for evidence of asymmetry (e.g. palpebral fissures, drooping of the angle of the mouth, loss of nasolabial fold) or abnormal movements (e.g. tics, dyskinesia, myokymia, fasciculations). Power of the facial muscles is tested by asking the patient (i) to elevate the eyebrows by looking upwards, and observing the corrugation of the forehead; (ii) to close the eyes firmly, and observing whether the eyelashes are buried equally on both sides after which the examiner should attempt to open the eyelids against resistance; (iii) to smile broadly, observing the depth of the nasolabial folds.

All three sections of the facial nerve should be tested in this manner since the upper face is relatively spared by an upper motor neurone lesion. An upper motor neurone source of lower facial weakness can usually be confirmed by inducing the patient to laugh or smile spontaneously (if a feeble joke does not produce this effect, the examiner may have to resort to tickling) in which case the smile becomes symmetrical.

Sensory

The nervus intermedius can be tested by applying a bent pin to the posterior aspect of the external auditory canal. Sensation in this area may be diminished (Hitzelberger's sign) in early compression of the seventh nerve, by acoustic neuroma for example, but this sign has not proved reliable in our hands.

Taste

Taste can be tested by applying a salty or sweet solution to the anterior two-thirds of each side of the protruded tongue in turn. Taste fibres travel with the lingual nerve but cross to the facial nerve in the chorda tympani so that taste is impaired if the facial nerve is compromised proximal to the junction with the chorda tympani (as it often is in Bell's palsy).

Reflexes

Corneal reflex and glabella tap sign as described under cranial nerve V. In frontal lobe lesions, contraction of the orbicularis oris may follow percussion of the closed lips (pouting response).

Cranial nerve VIII (acoustic and vestibular nerves)

Acoustic (auditory) nerve

Hearing is tested grossly by blocking one ear with a finger while the threshold of the other ear is determined by whispered or spoken voice at varying intensities. Normally the whispered word can be heard at a distance of about 60 cm. If one ear is deaf, the nature of the deafness is determined by two clinical tests after ensuring that the external auditory meatus is not obstructed.

Rinné test   The base of a vibrating tuning fork (128, 256, or 512 Hz) is placed on one mastoid process until it can no longer be heard. The vibrating prongs are then held next to the ear. If the tone is then audible, 'air conduction' (AC) is said to be better heard than 'bone conduction' (BC), which is normally so and is the case in mild perceptive (nerve) deafness. BC is better than AC in conduction deafness (due to external or middle ear disease). In severe nerve deafness the sound may be conducted through bone to the normal ear, thus giving a spurious result.

Weber's test   The base of a vibrating tuning fork is placed on the middle of the forehead. The sound is heard better on the normal side in the case of nerve deafness but is referred to the deaf ear in the case of conduction deafness (because of the lack of competing auditory stimuli through the normal channels).

It must be borne in mind that tuning fork tests use frequencies lower than those of the normal conversational range and that they are highly fallible. Audiometry is recommended in any case of deafness (see Chapter 9).

Vestibular nerve

There is no satisfactory bedside test for the vestibular nerves which are assessed by caloric testing and electronystagmography as described in Chapter 9. Positional vertigo and nystagmus may be sought by lowering the patient's head backwards over the end of the examination couch, first to one side, then to the other (Chapter 9).

Cranial nerves IX (glossopharyngeal), X (vagus) and XI (central part of the accessory nerve)

Motor

Observe quality of speech and coughing for dysphonia, from weakness of closure of the vocal cords (paralysis of vagus or its recurrent laryngeal branch), or for a nasal intonation from palatal weakness. Look at the posterior pharynx for unswallowed saliva and check swallowing while the patient drinks a glass of water. Movement of the palate is observed (i) during voluntary activity with the patient saying 'ah'; (ii) during reflex activity after touching the posterior pharyngeal wall with a wooden probe or tongue depressor ('gag reflex').

If both voluntary and reflex movement are impaired bilaterally (bulbar palsy), or the palate fails to elevate on one side, the lesion is of the lower motor neurone. If the palate cannot be elevated voluntarily but moves normally in the gag reflex, the lesion involves the upper motor neurone ('pseudobulbar palsy').

Sensory

The posterior pharyngeal wall is innervated by the glossopharyngeal nerve and sensation is tested by means of a wooden probe (a pin is too unkind) first on one side then the other.

Reflex

The gag reflex is described above. The cough reflex is usually not tested.

Cranial nerve XI (spinal part of the accessory nerve, arising from cervical cord segments 1–5)

This is solely motor, supplying the upper trapezius and the sternomastoid muscles. Its integrity is tested by instructing the patient to shrug the shoulders upwards against the pressure of the examiner's hand and to turn the head firmly against pressure while the sternomastoid muscles are palpated. Wasting and weakness of the affected muscles are noted.

Cranial nerve XII (hypoglossal nerve)

The patient protrudes the tongue and then pushes it into one cheek and then the other against pressure from the examiner's hand. With a unilateral lesion of the lower motor neurone, the tongue deviates to the side of the lesion (since the action of the hyoglossus muscle is to pull the tongue forwards), and pressure exerted against the cheek is diminished on the affected side. Slight deviation of the tongue may be seen with an upper motor neurone lesion, but in this case the deviation is to the side of the hemiparesis; i.e. opposite to the side of the lesion. Wasting and fasciculation of the tongue may be noted on the side of the lesion, or bilaterally in the case of bulbar palsy. Since a tremor may develop in a protruded tongue and obscure fasciculations, these are best sought with the tongue at rest on the floor of the mouth. Coarse undulations of the tongue musculature (myokymia) may be observed with central lesions such as brainstem gliomas.

Motor system (see also Chapter 3)

Inspection

The patient, wearing the minimum of clothing compatible with age and sex, lies comfortably on an examination couch in the supine position. The following are closely observed:

(a) Posture and development of the trunk and limbs. Symmetry of the upper limbs is checked. Shortening of one forearm by more than 1 cm suggests some disturbance of the opposite hemisphere (parietal region) at birth or in early childhood. Asymmetry of the hands, fingernails and of the lower limbs may provide supporting evidence. The patient then holds both arms in front of the body and closes the eyes while the examiner observes whether either arm drifts downwards from the horizontal level. This is a quick check of pyramidal, proprioceptive and cerebellar function since all are required to maintain posture. The lower limbs are similarly inspected. Pes cavus may suggest a congenital anomaly, such as spina bifida, or an hereditary disorder such as a spinocerebellar degeneration or peroneal muscular atrophy (Charcot-Marie-Tooth disease).

(b) Any involuntary movements.

(c) The degree and distribution of any muscular wasting.

(d) The presence of any muscular fasciculation.

Muscle tone

'Muscle tone' does not refer to the firmness or flabbiness of the muscle bellies but to the activity of the stretch reflexes, usually assessed by the resistance encountered on stretching the muscle at increasing velocities.

Diminished muscle tone may be inferred from posture. If the patient's elbows are resting on a firm base with the forearms held vertically, the wrist usually assumes a resting posture at an angle of about 30° above the horizontal line. If muscle tone is diminished (hypotonia), the wrist is held at or below the horizontal level. One foot may be seen to rest on a lower level than the other if that limb is hypotonic.

Muscle tone in the upper limbs is examined by passively flexing and extending the elbows and the wrists, and by pronating and supinating the wrists. If the patient has been noticed not to swing one arm on walking (as in Parkinson's disease), the tone of the shoulder muscle should be examined by rotary movements at the shoulder joint. The cogwheel rigidity of Parkinson's disease may be enhanced by asking the patient to make a mental calculation, clench the jaw, turn the head from side to side or to clench the fist on the opposite side. Muscle tone in the lower limbs is assessed by passively flexing and extending the hip, knee and ankle joints at varying velocities. Changes in muscle tone (hypotonia in disorders of the lower motor neurone and cerebellum; hypertonia in upper motor neurone lesions or Parkinson's disease) are discussed in Chapter 3.

Power

The examination of muscle power is best conducted in an orderly sequence, proceeding from proximal to distal muscles, testing abductors before adductors and flexor groups before extensors, so that any pattern of weakness becomes apparent while the examination is in progress. This is of particular importance in detecting an upper motor neurone ('pyramidal') pattern of weakness in which the flexors of the lower limbs (including the dorsiflexors of the ankles as part of the flexor synergy) are preferentially impaired. The exact manner in which each muscle group is most easily tested is best learned at the bedside and requires considerable practice so that the examination is carried out rapidly and accurately. When testing the power of the hip flexors it is helpful to keep one hand under the heel of the opposite foot. If the patient is not trying hard to flex the hip (because of pain, malingering or hysteria), normal counter pressure is not felt on the opposite side (Hoover's sign).

Muscle power may be graded on the MRC (Medical Research Council, United Kingdom) scale for progress assessment:

0   no movement
1   a flicker is perceptible in the muscle
2   the muscle can move the limb if the force of gravity is eliminated by supporting the limb
3   the muscle can elevate the limb against the force of gravity
4   the muscle can move the limb against resistance supplied by the examiner
5   normal power

The problem with the MRC scale is that most muscular weakness falls between 4 and 5 so that one has to resort to the cumbersome intermediate gradings of 4.25, 4.5 and 4.75.

If weakness of the lower limbs extends upwards to the trunk, the upper limit of motor deficit can sometimes be ascertained by asking the patient to try to sit up without using the arms. If the umbilicus deviates upwards, it indicates that the lower abdominal muscles are weaker than the upper (lesion around the T10 level). If expansion of the thoracic cage on deep inspiration is less in the lower part of the chest than the upper, it suggests that the lesion lies at the T5/6 level.

Reflexes

Tendon jerks

A brisk reflex contraction of most muscles can be obtained by tapping their tendons (or a bony attachment) with a percussion hammer so that the muscle is vibrated or transiently stretched, thus stimulating the primary endings of the muscle spindle. An afferent volley set up by percussion then traverses the monosynaptic arc, causing a reflex contraction (Fig. 3.4). This is a means of testing the integrity and excitability of various segmental levels in the spinal cord.

The patient lies supine with the upper limbs flexed, the elbows being supported on the examination couch and the forearms and hands resting lightly across the abdomen. The percussion hammer is lightly flicked from one radial styloid process to the other so that the amplitude of the reflex on each side may be compared. The biceps jerk is tested by tapping each biceps tendon separately. Then each arm is gently drawn across the abdomen to make the triceps tendon taut so that the triceps jerk may be tested. To elicit the finger jerk, the patient lightly clenches his fingers against the examiner's fingers so that tapping the examiner's fingers with the percussion hammer will transmit a vibration wave or brief stretch to the patient's finger flexors, which thus evokes the finger jerk. If the thumb is noted to flex with the fingers, this thumb reflex is known as Hoffman's sign. Hoffman's sign is traditionally elicited by flipping the terminal phalanx of the index or middle finger which transmits a similar vibratory stimulus to the tendons of finger and thumb flexors to that evoked by percussion of the fingers. Hoffman's sign is found whenever reflexes are brisk and is not specific for an upper motor neurone lesion.

To test knee jerks it is easiest to place one hand under both knees, lifting so that the lower limbs are partly flexed at the knees and the percussion hammer can be flicked from one ligamentum patellae to the other, to detect any asymmetry of knee jerks. The ankle jerks are most simply tested with the lower limbs abducted at the hips and the knees flexed, a position like the frog-kick in swimming breaststroke. The foot is then grasped by the examiner, moved rapidly up and down to ensure that the muscle is relaxed, then placed in the mid-position before the tendo Achillis is tapped. These minor points of technique are important because the reflex will not be detected if the patient is voluntarily holding the ankle rigidly in position, *or* if the tendon is so slack that the vibration from percussion is not transmitted, *or* if the ankle is sharply dorsiflexed so that the calf muscle is stretched so much that the ankle jerk is reflexly inhibited.

If reflexes are brisk, repetitive discharge of the stretch reflex arc (clonus) may be demonstrated by maintaining the appropriate muscle on stretch.

Superficial reflexes

These are best considered as protective reflexes by which stimulation of the skin induces a contraction of the underlying or surrounding muscles (comparable with the corneal reflex).

Abdominal reflexes

A pin is drawn briskly but lightly across the four quadrants of the abdomen in sequence, from outside inwards, running down along the line of the dermatomes. The stroke should not be so firm as to scarify the abdomen. The abdominal muscles are seen to contract in response to the stimulus.

Cremasteric reflexes

A brisk stroke on the inner side of the thigh produces contraction of the cremasteric muscle, causing the testis to retract.

Bulbocavernosus reflex

A sharp squeeze or gentle pinprick applied to the glans penis induces a contraction in the bulbocavernosus muscle which can be felt in the perineum at the base of the penis.

Anal reflex

A stroke or pinprick in the circumanal region induces contraction of the external sphincter which can be seen (or felt by a finger per rectum). The bulbocavernosus and anal reflexes are important to test in patients with sphincter disturbance, impotence or other symptoms suggesting a cauda equina or conus lesion.

Plantar responses

The lateral aspect of the sole (S1 dermatome) is stimulated by a firm stroke with a blunt object and the movement of the great toe is observed. The normal response of adults and children over the age of 12 months is flexion of the great toe (flexor plantar response). If flexor reflexes are released by damage to corticoreticulospinal pathways, as happens in most upper motor neurone lesions, the great toe extends as it does normally in infancy. Extension of the great toe (extensor plantar response, 'upgoing toe', or Babinski response) is often accompanied by abduction of the other toes. Although the movement of the great toe is extension in anatomical terms, it is part of a flexor protective reflex in physiological terms. This can be clearly seen in patients with an upper motor neurone lesion of the spinal cord (which releases flexor reflexes from brainstem control), in which case repeated stroking of the sole causes first a Babinski response, then dorsiflexion of the ankle as well, then flexion of the entire lower limb which becomes more marked with each stroke of the sole (flexor spasms).

The presence and the briskness of reflexes is indicated by the following symbols:

0 or —	absent
+	diminished
++	normal
+++	increased
++++	clonus present

Normal reflexes, the segments that mediate them and the way in which they are recorded, are listed in Table 2.1. The jaw jerk is included here because it is of relevance to the level of an upper motor neurone lesion, but other cranial nerve reflexes have been omitted.

Table 2.1   Normal reflexes

Reflexes		Response		Segments
Jaw		++		Cr n. 5
		right	left	
Biceps		++	++	C 5–6
Radial (brachioradialis, 'supinator')		++	++	C 5–6
Triceps		++	++	C 7
Finger		++	++	C 8
Abdominal	upper	++	++	T 9–10
	lower	++	++	T 11–12
Cremasteric		++	++	L 1, 2
Knee		++	++	L 3–4
Extensor hallucis		++	++	L 5
Ankle		++	++	S 1
Plantar		↓	↓	S 1
Bulbocavernosus		++	++	S 2–3–4
Anal		++	++	S 3–4–5

An extensor plantar response is indicated by reversed arrows. Primitive reflexes released in frontal lobe disorders include pouting and sucking responses, grasp reflexes and the palmar-mental response (contraction of the chin muscles ipsilateral to a firm stroke across the thenar eminence).

Coordination

If position sense and motor pathways are intact, coordination tests assess cerebellar function (see also Chapter 10).

Upper limbs

The following tests of coordination are commonly used:
(a) Rhythmic repetitive movements, such as tapping the fingers rapidly on a table or other surface. Dysrhythmia may be heard as well as seen.
(b) Alternating movements, such as tapping the opposite hand or thigh with pronation-supination of the wrist. If speed decreases and amplitude of hand movement increases as the alternating movement continues, this is known as dysdiadochokinesia.

(c) Rebound phenomenon. The patient is asked to elevate the extended arms briskly in front of the body and halt them in a given position. In cerebellar disorders, the movement is slow to start and slow to stop so that the affected limb shoots past the intended end-point (rebound phenomenon).

(d) Finger-nose test. The patient is asked to touch the tip of his nose, then touch the examiner's finger which is held in front of the patient, then to touch his own nose again. The movement should be performed slowly, then rapidly, to bring out any possible defect. Abnormalities that may be noted are: (i) Dysmetria. The finger falls short of the target or exceeds it (past-pointing) or deviates to one side or the other (usually to the side of a cerebellar lesion). (ii) Action tremor. A tremor accompanies the movement throughout its duration. Action tremor is not of cerebellar origin and must not be confused with intention tremor. (iii) Intention tremor. The amplitude of tremor increases as the target is approached.

Lower limbs

(a) Rapid tapping movement of the feet.
(b) Heel-knee-shin test. The patient lifts one leg, then places it on the knee and runs it down the shin of the other leg.
(c) Toe-finger test. The patient lifts his leg so as to touch the examiner's finger, which is moved from point to point. Intention tremor may be seen.

In cases of cerebellar disturbance, certain features may have been noted earlier in the examination.
(a) Posture. The head may be held on one side with the occiput to the side of the lesion.
(b) Gait. The patient may walk with a wide base and turn in a series of steps ('by numbers'), a form of decomposition of movement, or may deviate to the side of the lesion. When asked to walk on the spot with the eyes closed, the patient rotates to the side of the lesion.
(c) Hypotonia of the affected side. If the knee jerk is tested when the patient is sitting on the examination couch with the legs suspended, the leg may swing to and fro after the reflex contraction, an undamped or 'pendular' knee jerk.
(d) Nystagmus.
(e) Dysarthria.

Sensory system (see also Chapter 4)

Various forms of sensibility may be tested.

Light touch

Touch with a wisp of cotton wool is used as the testing stimulus.

Pain sensation

Superficial pain sensation is tested by pricking the skin with a pin. The patient may be asked to distinguish the sensation elicited by the sharp and blunt ends of the pin.

Temperature sensation

A cold object is applied to the skin and the sensation of coldness experienced from different areas is compared by the patient. An elaboration of this test is to use test tubes filled with water at 7°C above and below the skin temperature, so that the patient can detect the difference between heat and cold in various areas.

Proprioception

This is often called 'joint position sense' but also depends on muscle afferent fibres. It is tested by asking patients (with eyes closed) to state the direction of movement taking place at a joint when it is passively moved by the examiner. Movements at distal joints of toes and fingers are commonly tested but, if proprioceptive loss is gross, movement at wrist or elbow, ankle or knee may have to be tested. If the upper limbs can be maintained in a constant outstretched posture without drifting away and without unintended movements of the fingers, it is unlikely that formal examination will discern any proprioceptive loss in the upper limbs.

Vibration sense

This is examined by placing the base of the vibrating tuning fork (128 Hz) on bony prominences such as the terminal interphalangeal joints of fingers and toes. Normally, vibration sense is preserved at these distal joints but if not it should be tested at more proximal joints such as ankles, knees, wrists and elbows.

Two-point discrimination

The pulps of the finger should be able to distinguish two points separated by 3 mm and the sole of the foot can do so if separation of the points is increased to 3 cm.

Stereognosis

The ability to distinguish the size or texture of small objects is tested by placing coins or various materials in each hand while the patient's eyes are closed.

Figure writing (Graphaesthesia)

A test of fine sensibility similar to stereognosis is to trace on the patient's skin a figure between 1 and 9, which should be identified by the patient with eyes closed.

In practice, these tests are not necessarily all employed in examination of every patient. Sensory testing is guided by the history. If the patient has experienced paraesthesiae or numbness in a certain area, that area is tested first and compared with the nearest adjacent normal area. The pin or other testing object is then advanced from the area of sensory impairment toward the normal area until a line of demarcation is reached where sensation becomes normal. In this way, the distribution of sensory loss can be mapped rapidly and determined to be of peripheral, spinal root, spinal cord or cerebral origin.

General examination

Other systems should also be examined in the normal way with particular emphasis on examination of the pulse, heart, abdomen and lymph glands. The blood pressure must always be recorded, in both lying and standing positions if there have been symptoms of postural hypotension. The radial pulses are asymmetrical in subclavian stenosis and a bruit may be heard above the clavicle. The blood pressure should be recorded in each arm separately in patients with suspected cerebral vascular insufficiency. The texture of the skin, distribution of body hair, testicular size and breast development are indicators of pituitary function which may be impaired by tumours in or near the pituitary gland or by a longstanding increase in intracranial pressure. Testicular atrophy is found in dystrophia myotonia.

Reference

Aids to the Examination of the Peripheral Nervous System. (1986) London, Baillière-Tindall.

3 Motor System

Functional division of motor pathways

The motor system may be considered in terms of five main functional divisions — the lower motor neurone (final common pathway), the pyramidal (corticospinal tract), extrapyramidal tracts, cerebellum and cerebral cortex (Fig. 3.1).

Lower motor neurone

The lower motor neurone consists of a motor unit which comprises an anterior horn cell (motoneurone) with an axon that divides to supply 100–200 muscle fibres (Fig. 3.8) that all contract when the motor unit is active. The force of contraction depends on the number of active motoneurones and their rate of firing (up to about 100/s). Disorders of the lower motor neurone involve the motor unit, e.g. poliomyelitis and motor neurone disease (affecting anterior horn cells), intervertebral disc protrusions (which may compress motor roots), plexus lesions and peripheral neuropathies. The motor unit may also be affected by failure of neuromuscular transmission (myasthenia gravis) or disorders of muscle fibres (myopathies).

The pyramidal (corticospinal) tract

This arises chiefly, but not exclusively, from the precentral gyrus of the cerebral cortex, and crosses in the pyramids at the lower end of the medulla. The descending fibres terminate directly, or through an interconnecting neurone, on the anterior horn cells (Fig. 3.2). A pure pyramidal tract lesion is rarely seen because the tract is accompanied throughout its course by an extrapyramidal pathway consisting of corticoreticulospinal fibres, interruption of which causes increased muscle tone (spasticity). Disorders involving the corticospinal tract (and accompanying corticoreticulospinal fibres) are spoken of clinically as *upper motor neurone lesions*. Such disorders are very common and are seen, for example, after strokes or injuries involving the spinal cord.

Fig. 3.1 Diagram of upper and lower motor neurones, showing the levels of the nervous system at which they may be affected and the distribution of weakness that results. The pyramidal tract is accompanied by cortico-reticulospinal fibres (interrupted lines), damage to which causes spasticity. (From Lance and McLeod, 1981, with permission of Butterworths, London.)

Extrapyramidal tracts

Descending pathways other than the pyramidal tract are connected with the spinal motoneurone pool, mainly through interneurones, and play a role in voluntary movement (Fig. 11.1). These arise from the fronto-parietal cortex, basal ganglia, cerebellum and other nuclei in the brainstem and, after interconnections, finally project downstream as rubro-spinal, reticulospinal and vestibulospinal pathways. *Extrapyramidal disorders* are manifested chiefly as abnormalities of muscle tone, posture and movement. A common example is Parkinson's disease.

Fig. 3.2 Pathways of corticospinal tracts. F, face; A, arm; T, trunk; L, leg.

Cerebellum

The cerebellum has reciprocal connections with sensorimotor cortex, reticular formation, vestibular nuclei and spinal cord (Figs 10.3–10.5). It participates in the programming of ballistic (rapid) movement and feedback control of ramp (slow) movements. Cerebellar disorders are characterized by hypotonia, incoordination and ataxia.

Cerebral cortex

At the highest level, damage to certain areas of the cerebral cortex, which in some way coordinate thought and action, may impair or prevent willed movement. These disorders are known as *apraxias*. For example, in an ideational apraxia which follows damage to the dominant parietal lobe, a movement cannot be performed as instructed although the appropriate motor pathways are intact.

Reflexes

Reflex activity plays a prominent part in the maintenance of posture and the execution of movement.

The simplest reflex is the stretch reflex (Fig. 3.3). The *muscle spindle*, the stretch receptor in muscle, consists of nuclear bag and nuclear chain endings whose afferents are Group Ia and II fibres. The muscle spindle (with its intrafusal fibres) lies parallel to the extrafusal muscle fibres. When the muscle spindle is stretched, impulses pass along Group Ia afferent fibres which synapse monosynaptically with *alpha motoneurones*. These in turn discharge, causing the muscle to contract. Group II muscle

Fig. 3.3 Stretch reflex arc. Group Ia afferent fibres, connected to the primary spindle endings, synapse directly with alpha motoneurones in the anterior horn, whose axons innervate the extrafusal muscle fibres. Group Ib afferent fibres are connected to Golgi tendon organs. Group II afferent fibres connected to secondary spindle endings are mainly inhibitory on extensor motoneurones and facilitatory on flexor motoneurones. The gamma motoneurones innervate the muscle spindle. Descending motor pathways (corticospinal, reticulospinal, vestibulospinal) regulate alpha and gamma motoneurone excitability.

afferents from muscle spindles exert mainly inhibitory effects on extensor motoneurones and facilitatory effects on flexor motoneurones, i.e. they act as flexor reflex afferents (FRA) and this reflex action becomes apparent in spasticity. *Golgi tendon organs* lie near tendons and are connected to Ib afferents; these are highly sensitive to active contraction and also to sudden increase in tension. *Gamma motoneurones* which innervate the muscle spindle and regulate its sensitivity to stretch, also lie in the anterior horn of the spinal cord. Their action during movement is to cause contraction of the muscle spindle fibres so that afferents can continue to act as sensors during contraction when the extrafusal fibres shorten.

Supraspinal control of alpha and gamma motoneurones is derived from corticospinal, vestibulospinal, reticulospinal and rubrospinal pathways (Fig. 3.3).

Tendon reflexes

Clinically the reflex arc is tested by way of the tendon or stretch reflexes. A brisk tap over the tendon or a vibration wave induced by percussion of bone to which the tendon attaches, stretches the muscle spindle and excites the monosynaptic reflex causing the extrafusal fibres to contract (Fig. 3.4). This is an example of a *phasic stretch reflex* in which there is excitation from a more or less synchronous afferent volley.

Fig. 3.4 Mechanism of a tendon reflex. A brisk tap with a percussion hammer stretches the tendon (1), and the muscle spindle (2), initiating a volley of impulses in the Group Ia afferent fibres that excites the alpha motoneurone thus causing the extrafusal fibres to contract (3).

Table 3.1   Commonly tested tendon reflexes

Reflex	Segment
Jaw jerk	5th cranial nerve (motor nerve)
Biceps jerk	C5, 6
Brachioradialis (supinator) jerk	C5, 6
Triceps jerk	C7
Finger-flexion reflex	C8
Knee jerk	L3, 4
Ankle jerk	S1

Reflexes that are commonly tested clinically and the segments through which they operate are shown in Table 3.1.

Alteration in tendon reflexes

Tendon jerks vary in amplitude from person to person but are normally symmetrical.

Depression of reflex activity   Reflexes may be depressed because of impairment of function of parts of the reflex arc.

Muscle spindle — selective damage to muscle spindles is not known clinically. They do not share in the muscular atrophy of motor neurone disease.

Gamma motoneurone — fusimotor activity may be depressed in spinal shock and probably in acute cerebellar lesions. As a result, the muscle spindle becomes less sensitive to stretch.

Afferent fibres — e.g. peripheral neuropathy, dorsal root lesions.

Anterior horn cells — e.g. poliomyelitis, motor neurone disease.

Efferent fibres — e.g. peripheral neuropathy, ventral root lesions.

Muscles — e.g. myopathy.

Contraction of antagonists — e.g. poor relaxation, extrapyramidal rigidity.

Exaggeration of reflex activity   The most common pathological cause of increased tendon reflexes is an upper motor neurone lesion, but they may also be exaggerated as a result of anxiety, after exercise and in thyrotoxicosis.

Reinforcement of reflexes

Reflex activity may be heightened by *reinforcement*, e.g. a depressed biceps jerk may become brisker if the patient is asked to squeeze an object hard with the opposite hand at the time the reflex is being elicited, or lower limb reflexes may be enhanced by the patient pulling one hand against the other (Jendrassik manoeuvre).

Reflexes should not be considered absent unless reinforcement has been attempted. The effort increases alpha motoneurone activity in the spinal cord and thus increases the sensitivity of the stretch reflex.

Spread of reflexes

Sometimes in normal people, and frequently in patients with upper motor neurone disease, one sees what is known as a *spread of reflexes*. For example, if one elicits a supinator jerk, the biceps and triceps as well as the brachioradialis may contract briskly in response to the tap over the radius.

This is due to alpha motoneurone hyperexcitability and spreading of a wave of vibration that excites muscle spindles in distant muscles causing them to contract reflexly (Fig. 3.5). Primary endings in muscle spindles are very sensitive to vibration.

Tonic reflexes

Tonic reflexes (as distinct from phasic reflexes) are those that are excited by a sustained asynchronous afferent stimulus. In cats, there is some evidence that different alpha motoneurones subserve the phasic and tonic reflexes but there is no evidence that this is so in man. Tonic stretch reflexes become apparent in normal people during anxiety and postural adjustment or voluntary muscle contraction. They cannot usually be detected in relaxed normal human subjects. They are increased in upper motor neurone lesions (spasticity) and some extrapyramidal disorders (rigidity). Application of a vibrator to the muscle belly or tendon elicits a tonic reflex contraction in man (tonic vibration reflex or TVR), that has some application in physiotherapy.

Superficial cutaneous reflexes

These are polysynaptic reflexes, that are often relayed through more than one segment (Table 3.2).

Muscle tone

Muscle tone is a clinical term used to describe the resistance of muscles to passive movement. The resistance is determined partly by mechanical

Fig. 3.5 The radial ('supinator') jerk. Percussion of the radius initiates a vibration wave which stimulates primary spindle endings as it traverses muscle bellies, causing a reflex contraction (+) of biceps, triceps, brachioradialis, finger flexors and extensors. The limb moves in the direction of the stronger muscles so that the elbow and fingers flex, the reaction of a normal 'supinator' or radial jerk. Multiple muscle contractions are observed more clearly in upper motor neurone lesions, a finding termed 'reflex irradiation'. (From Lance and McLeod, 1981, with permission of Butterworths, London.)

Table 3.2   Polysynaptic reflexes that are often relayed through more than one segment

Reflex	Segment
Corneal	Cranial nerves V and VII
Abdominal	
Upper	T9, 10
Lower	T11, 12
Cremasteric	L1, 2
Plantar	S1
Bulbocavernosus	S2, 3, 4
Anal	S3, 4, 5

factors (joints, ligaments and viscoelastic properties of muscle) and partly by reflex contraction of the muscle (the tonic stretch reflex).

Tone will be decreased when there is an interruption of the stretch reflex arc, such as may occur in peripheral neuropathies and other lower motor neurone disorders. Tone is also decreased in cerebellar disorders and immediately after spinal cord injuries (spinal shock), probably as a result of decreased responsiveness of the muscle spindle to stretch, consequent upon a depression of fusimotor activity.

Tone is increased in upper motor neurone disorders, when it increases in proportion to the velocity of the stretch ('spasticity'). It is also increased in certain extrapyramidal disorders such as Parkinson's disease, when it is less sensitive to the velocity of stretch and is usually interrupted by tremor mechanisms ('cog-wheel rigidity'). *Dystonia* is the term used to describe a transient or persistent increase in tone that is associated with co-contraction of antagonistic muscles and assumption of abnormal posture.

Lower motor neurone disorders

Lower motor neurone disorders may result from disease or damage to the anterior horn cell, motor root or peripheral nerve (see Figs 3.1 and 3.8).

(a) Anterior horn cells, e.g. poliomyelitis, motor neurone disease, syringomyelia.

(b) Motor roots, e.g. cervical or lumbar disc protrusions, malignancy.

(c) Peripheral nerve, e.g. Bell's palsy, nerve injuries, peripheral neuropathy.

Clinical features of lower motor neurone disorders

Muscle weakness

This may range from slight weakness (paresis) to total paralysis.

Muscle wasting

Peripheral nerve lesions result in muscle wasting and weakness in the appropriate distribution of the damaged nerve. Root injuries result in wasting that follows a segmental distribution. Anterior horn cell disease may give rise to diffuse weakness and wasting.

Fig. 3.6 Electromyogram recorded on maximum voluntary effort from (a) normal muscle, (b) denervated muscle, (c) muscular dystrophy. Time marker: 5 ms intervals. Calibration 2 mV (a+c), 5 mV (b).

Fasciculation

Coarse fascicular twitches, caused by spontaneous contractions of one or more motor units, are seen in lower motor neurone disorders, especially in chronic degenerative disease of the anterior horn cell, such as motor neurone disease. *Benign fasciculations* can occur in normal people especially if the muscle is in a state of tension. Benign fasciculations are coarse, and can usually be seen to affect the same fascicle repeatedly. Pathological fasciculations due to degeneration of nerves or nerve cells are an irregular twitching seen in various parts of a relaxed muscle; minutes may elapse before the same fascicle contracts for a second time. Fasciculation has pathological significance only when the muscle concerned is atrophied or weak.

A related phenomenon is *myokymia*, an irregular undulation of superficial muscle fibres. It commonly occurs around the eye and is usually benign but persistent facial or limb myokymia may be a sign of involvement of the appropriate efferent pathway.

Fibrillation is an electromyographic term and refers to spontaneous electrical activity in individual muscle fibres after denervation (Fig. 3.7).

Fig. 3.7 Spontaneous fibrillation, recorded through a concentric needle electrode from a denervated muscle. (Time marker, 5 ms intervals.)

Hypotonia

Tonic stretch reflexes are diminished in proportion to the degree of muscular weakness.

Tendon reflexes

These are depressed in proportion to the degree of damage to the efferent limb of the reflex arc. They may, however, be increased if there is an associated upper motor neurone lesion (e.g. motor neurone disease).

Contractures

Progressive shortening of muscle bellies in paralysed muscles or in their antagonists may result in deformities of the limb (contractures).

Trophic changes

These are partly a result of disuse, and partly a result of vasomotor (autonomic) involvement. The skin is cold, cyanosed, smooth and dry. Toe-nails, finger-nails and bones become brittle.

Electromyogram (EMG)

The features of denervation are spontaneous fibrillation, positive sharp waves, a reduced pattern of motor unit activity on maximum voluntary effort and polyphasic, large amplitude motor units of long duration (Figs 3.6, 3.7).

Disorders of the neuromuscular junction and muscles

Failure of neuromuscular transmission causes fatiguability and weakness of muscles, and is seen most commonly in myasthenia gravis. Disease of muscle fibres (myopathy) causes wasting and weakness of

Fig. 3.8 Lower motor neurone. Lower motor neurone disorders may result from diseases of (1) the anterior horn cell, (2) motor roots, or (3) peripheral nerve. Disorders of the neuromuscular junction (4) and muscle fibres (5) may stimulate lower motor neurone lesions by affecting the distal parts of the motor unit.

muscles. Muscular dystrophies are genetically determined myopathies.

Clinical features

Muscle weakness   In myopathies, muscle weakness is usually proximal and may be restricted to particular muscle groups. In myasthenia gravis, the characteristic feature is weakness after sustained or repeated effort (muscle fatiguability); extraocular, bulbar, and proximal limb muscles are most commonly affected.

Muscle wasting   Muscle wasting may be severe in myopathies, but is not a feature of myasthenia gravis. In myopathies, muscle wasting and weakness may be restricted to particular muscle groups, especially proximal muscles.

Fasciculation   Absent.

Hypotonia   Tone is reduced in proportion to the degree of muscle weakness.

Reflexes   Reflexes are depressed when muscle wasting is advanced, but may not be affected in the early stages since muscle spindles are spared.

Contractures   Contractures occur in wasted muscles.

Trophic changes   Trophic changes may be seen in paralysed limbs.

EMG   The electromyographic features of myopathies are a full pattern of activity on maximum voluntary effort with short duration polyphasic units of reduced amplitude (Fig. 3.6).

Upper motor neurone disorders

The descriptive terms 'upper motor neurone disorder', 'pyramidal tract disorder' and 'corticospinal tract disorder' are all used synonymously in clinical medicine. This is not an accurate use of terms in an anatomical or physiological sense, but it is hallowed by tradition. Pure pyramidal tract lesions are rarely seen clinically; accompanying corticoreticulospinal fibres are usually involved also.

The major contribution to the pyramidal tract in man arises from the precentral and postcentral gyri, and from the paracentral lobule, with significant contributions from areas 5, 6 and 7 (Fig. 3.9). Only 2-3% of the fibres arise from Betz cells.

The corticospinal and corticobulbar fibres have a definite topographical distribution (Fig. 3.10). At the lowermost part of the precentral gyrus are the areas for larynx and pharynx, above which are the areas for palate, mandible and tongue, and then the centres for lower and upper face. The upper face has a bilateral representation like the pharynx and larynx and sternomastoid muscles. Lower limb areas lie in the upper part of the motor strip and paracentral lobule so that lesions in the parasagittal region (e.g. meningiomas), or sagittal sinus thrombosis, may cause lower limb paralysis with sparing of the upper limbs (Fig. 3.1). Conversely tumours and vascular lesions in the lower part of the motor strip may involve the opposite side of the face and upper limb exclusively.

The corticospinal and corticobulbar tracts descend in the corona radiata to the internal capsule, where they occupy mainly its posterior

Fig. 3.9 Origin of corticospinal tracts from cerebral cortex. Most of the fibres in the corticospinal tracts arise from the motor cortex (area 4), premotor cortex (area 6) and somatosensory cortex (areas 3, 1, 2). The supplementary motor cortex (area 8) plays an important part in programming movements. (Modified from D. Cogan. *Neurology of the Ocular Muscles*, 2nd edn, 1966, courtesy of Charles C. Thomas, Springfield, Illinois.)

Fig. 3.10 Topographical distribution of origin of corticospinal tracts from cerebral cortex (after Penfield).

limb; the fibres from the face and shoulder lie anteriorly, and those for the lower limb posteriorly (Fig. 3.2). The face and upper limb may be selectively paralysed by thrombosis of the recurrent branch of the anterior cerebral artery (Heubner's artery) which supplies the area of the internal capsule containing the relevant fibres.

In the midbrain, the corticospinal tract runs in the middle three-fifths of the cerebral peduncles; in the pons it becomes broken into scattered bundles by transverse fibres and by the pontine grey matter; in the medulla the fibres come together again to form the pyramids (Fig. 3.2). About 70–90% of the fibres cross in the decussation of the pyramids. Most of the uncrossed fibres run in the ventral corticospinal tract, and cross before terminating on the anterior horn cells chiefly of the neck and trunk muscles. Corticospinal tract fibres terminate on anterior horn cells either directly or through internuncial cells.

The pyramidal tract is not essential for most voluntary movements which can be carried out by primates after the pyramids have been sectioned. However, in contrast to the extrapyramidal motor system, it is responsible for fine and skilled movements, particularly of hands and fingers. It also has an inhibitory effect on antigravity muscles and promotes abduction of upper limbs and flexion of lower limbs, i.e. it breaks up the pattern of reflex standing in man (flexed upper limbs and extended lower limbs) which is determined mainly by extrapyramidal pathways.

Clinical features of upper motor neurone disorders

The commonest cause of an upper motor neurone disorder is a vascular lesion involving the internal capsule. This is the most common type of 'stroke' and since the corticospinal and corticobulbar fibres are close together in this region, they are all affected. This gives rise to a paralysis (hemiplegia) or weakness ('hemiparesis') of the opposite side of the body (Fig. 3.1). The main features of hemiplegia from any cerebral lesion, which should be contrasted with those of lower motor neurone disorders, are described below.

Muscle weakness

This always affects groups of muscles rather than individual muscles. Bilateral movements of jaws, upper face, neck, pharynx, larynx, thorax, and upper abdomen are little affected.

Ocular movements   Immediately after a lesion of the internal capsule, the eyes may deviate to the side of the lesion in an unconscious patient. In the conscious patient there may be weakness of conjugate deviation to the opposite side (see Chapter 9). This usually lasts for only a few hours or days and is rarely permanent.

Head and neck   As with the eyes, there may be a deviation of the head or neck to the side of the lesion in the comatose patient.

Face   The upper face is bilaterally innervated and is little affected. The lower face is weak but this may be apparent only as a filling-in of the nasolabial fold on the affected side or a slight drooping of the corner of the mouth. Movements of the face following emotional stimuli, e.g. laughing or crying, may be quite normal because they are effected through extrapyramidal connections.

Jaw, palate, tongue   Like other bilaterally innervated structures, these are only slightly affected. There may be transient weakness of these structures on the side opposite the lesion.

Limbs   The side opposite the lesion is weak; fine skilled movements of fingers and toes are most affected. In upper limbs, the abductors are primarily involved (deltoids, spinati, and finger abductors) and, in lower limbs, the flexors (hip flexors, hamstrings, dorsiflexors of ankle and toes).

Gait   The upper limb on the affected side is held flexed and adducted. There is difficulty in flexing the lower limbs, and it is necessary to circumduct the leg at the hip in order to bring the limb forward. The foot is plantar-flexed and the shoe drags along the ground.

Muscle wasting

Any muscular wasting results from disuse, except in the rare syndrome of wasting from a parietal lobe lesion, the mechanism of which is unknown.

Fasciculations

Fasciculations do not occur in upper neurone lesions.

Hypertonia

Immediately after a capsular lesion, the limbs may be completely flaccid. After 2-3 weeks, tone increases and the limbs are said to be spastic.

Increased resistance to passive movement is most pronounced in the adductors and internal rotators of the shoulder, the flexors of the elbow, wrist and fingers, and the pronators of the forearm. In the lower limb the resistance is greater in the adductors of the hip, extensors of the hip and knee, and plantar-flexors of the foot and toes. The hemiplegic posture is the result of the abnormal distribution of muscle tone. It is influenced by tonic neck and labyrinthine reflexes, disinhibited from cortical control, and represents the antigravity posture (decorticate posture) of reflex standing in man. Spasticity is caused by the release of anterior horn cells from tonic inhibition exerted by the corticoreticulospinal pathway.

The resistance to stretch seen in spasticity is velocity-dependent; i.e. the resistance is increased with faster stretching movements. Therefore in testing clinically for muscle tone all limbs should be moved through a range of velocities.

One of the features of spasticity of capsular hemiplegia is the 'clasp-knife' phenomenon seen in the extensor muscles of the lower limbs. Muscle tension increases with velocity of stretch to about the mid-position of a joint. The sudden relaxation of tension is considered to be caused by inhibition arising from activation of Group II afferent fibres by increasing muscle length, although the Golgi tendon organs may initially cause some inhibition through Group Ib afferents (Fig. 3.3). The limb remains hypotonic as long as the extensor muscle is stretched beyond the 'clasp-knife' point but spasticity becomes apparent again as soon as the limb is extended.

The increased muscle tone in upper motor neurone disorders is due to hyperexcitability of alpha motoneurones, which then become more readily excited reflexly by passive stretch. There is no direct evidence for hyperactivity of gamma motoneurones, which would theoretically cause the muscle spindles to become more responsive to stretch.

There is little increase in tone after section of the medullary pyramids in monkeys. The spasticity which follows upper motor neurone lesions in man is probably the consequence of damage to the extra-pyramidal corticoreticulospinal pathway which has an inhibitory influence on the spinal motor neurone pool.

Reflexes

After the initial stages of an acute capsular lesion the deep tendon reflexes become exaggerated, and 'clonus', a rhythmic series of contractions in response to maintained stretch, may be elicited.

The increased reflex activity can be explained on the basis of alpha motoneurone hyperactivity, which also accounts for irradiation or spread of reflexes and clonus.

The finger flexion reflex may be increased, and Hoffman's sign, (obtained by vibrating the tendons and muscles by flicking the terminal phalanx of a finger), which is merely another way of eliciting the thumb and finger flexion reflex, may also be positive. Abdominal and cremasteric reflexes are often, but not invariably, lost.

The plantar reflex   Babinski (1896) was the first to establish the plantar response as one of the most important signs in clinical neurology. Until the age of 18 months, the great toe extends (dorsiflexes) in response to stimulation of the lateral aspect of the sole as part of an uncontrolled protective response which involves all the flexors of the lower limb (including extensor hallucis longus and other dorsiflexors of the feet and toes since they act physiologically as flexor muscles). When the infant learns to stand, flexor reflexes are inhibited from the brainstem by a reticulospinal pathway so that flexor pathways may be used for volitional movement such as walking. The great toe then plantar-flexes in response to stimulation of the sole (flexor plantar response or 'downgoing toe'). After damage to upper motor neurone pathways, flexor reflexes are released so that the toe extends (physiological flexion) if the sole is stroked (extensor plantar response, 'up-going toe' or Babinski response). In addition, there may be abduction (fanning) of the toes. In such pathological states, there is an increase in the receptive field of the reflex; it can sometimes be elicited from the skin of the tibial surface of the leg. The release of flexor reflexes may also give rise to *flexor spasms*, particularly if brainstem control of segmental mechanisms is impaired by a *spinal* lesion.

The following important points should be noted.
(a) The outer border of the sole of the foot (S1 dermatome) should be stimulated with a light stroke. The patient should be warned of the impending stimulus, and asked to relax.
(b) The Babinski reflex must be distinguished from a withdrawal response in which there is extension of the big toe associated with hip and knee flexion.
(c) The associated fanning of the toes may be of significance in confirming an isolated extensor plantar response.
(d) The extensor plantar response indicates what is termed clinically 'pyramidal tract disease'. However, it does not correlate completely with lesions of the anatomical corticospinal tracts. In other words, one can have corticospinal tract damage without a positive Babinski sign, and a positive Babinski sign without any corticospinal tract damage. It is an oversimplification to equate absolutely a positive Babinski sign with corticospinal tract disease, since it is caused by damage to corticoreticulospinal fibres controlling flexor reflexes. Positive Babinski responses

are found in the first 18 months of life, in sleep, in deep coma, and after epileptic seizures. In these conditions there is functional rather than structural impairment of the pathways.

Contractures

Contractures develop in longstanding upper motor neurone disorders if adequate physiotherapy is not instituted.

Trophic changes

These are inconspicuous.

Electromyogram

There are no signs of denervation.

Central motor conduction studies

A brisk muscular contraction can be induced by an electromagnetic, or a brief high voltage electrical stimulus applied to the human motor cortex through the intact scalp, and the latency of the response measured. If a similar response is elicited by stimulating the cervical cord, and its latency subtracted from that of the first response, central conduction time and velocity may be estimated.

References

Adams R.D. and Victor M. (1985) *Principles of Neurology*, 3rd edn. McGraw-Hill, New York.

Burke D. and Lance J.W. (1986) Function and dysfunction of the myotatic unit. In *Diseases of the Nervous System*, pp. 337–51. Eds A.K. Asbury, G.M. McKhann and W.I. McDonald. W.B. Saunders, Philadelphia.

Lance J.W. and McLeod J.G. (1981) *A Physiological Approach to Clinical Neurology*, 3rd edn. Butterworths, London.

4 Sensory System

The sensory system is usually considered and examined clinically as an entity separate from the motor system, but of course the two are closely related. Motor and reflex functions depend very much on the pattern of their sensory input. Clinical examples of this interdependence of the motor and the sensory system are inability to move a limb if all the dorsal roots are sectioned, and the disturbance of gait caused by an interruption of sensory pathways from the lower limbs. Most motor functions are ultimately an elaboration and integration of basic reflex mechanisms.

The examination of sensation

The patient's history is of considerable importance. For example, he or she may complain of feelings of 'pins and needles' (paraesthesiae), numbness, burning, coldness, tingling and electric shock sensations on bending the neck (Lhermitte's sign), and band-like constrictions (with spinal cord lesions). Patients may notice a difference in temperature sensation in their legs when they sit in a hot bath or in their two hands when they place them in hot water. Patients often use descriptive terms such as 'numbness' in a different sense to the doctor, and it is important to determine precisely what they mean.

When a patient complains of an abnormal sensation, one must determine its site; nature and quality; radiation; provoking and relieving factors; duration and time of onset; associated features, e.g. sweating, redness, dryness of skin, hyperalgesia.

Examination of the sensory system is the most difficult part of the neurological examination. Sensation is a purely subjective phenomenon and for accurate testing a fully conscious, alert, intelligent, cooperative patient (and doctor) is desirable. Such an ideal combination of qualities may not be present. It is important to avoid suggesting to the patient sensory changes which may not exist since many patients are highly suggestible. The key point is to relate the sensory examination to the clinical history. For example, if the patient complains of numbness in the little and ring fingers, the examination starts by comparing sensation in the presumed numb area with that of the index finger and thumb; the numb area is then delineated precisely by moving the pin or other test object from the abnormal to the normal area so that a clear end-point is obtained, and the distribution of sensory loss can be related to a peripheral nerve, spinal root, or central lesion. Similarly, if paraesthesiae are unilateral, one side of the body is compared with the other or, if the abnormal sensations are in the lower limbs, testing proceeds from below upwards to determine the upper level of sensory loss.

The sensations that are commonly tested clinically, as outlined in Chapter 2, are: (i) light touch, with a wisp of cotton wool; (ii) pain, with the point of a pin (the stimulus must be felt as sharp); (iii) temperature, with hot and cold objects; (iv) vibration sense, with a tuning fork of 128 Hz; (v) joint position sense; (vi) tactile discrimination, with compass points (usually < 3 mm on the fingers or < 3 cm on the feet; (vii) stereognosis, or the recognition of shape and form.

Pathways

Human cutaneous nerves

Human cutaneous nerves contain myelinated (A) fibres which range in diameter from about 2 to 16 μm and unmyelinated (C) fibres, all having their cell bodies in the dorsal root ganglia. They terminate peripherally in the skin and deeper structures as free nerve endings or encapsulated endings such as Meissner's corpuscles and Pacinian corpuscles. Some of these encapsulated endings are specially adapted to respond to certain stimuli, e.g. Pacinian corpuscles respond to displacement and vibration. Some receptors respond to more than one type of stimulus, e.g. some mechanoreceptors are sensitive to changes in temperature. The free nerve endings also play an important role in sensory discrimination, and are divided into three groups — mechanosensitive, thermosensitive and polymodal receptors.

Spinal cord

Pain fibres run for one or two segments in Lissauer's tract before entering the dorsal horn; small myelinated fibres synapse in Rexed laminae I and V and unmyelinated fibres synapse in lamina II (substantia gelatinosa) where substance P and other neuropeptides are transmitters (Fig. 4.1). They then cross to the opposite side of the spinal cord to join the lateral spinothalamic tract (Fig. 4.2). Proprioceptive afferents enter the

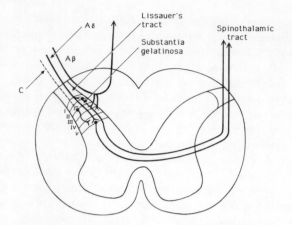

Fig. 4.1 Pathways of pain fibres in dorsal horn of spinal cord.

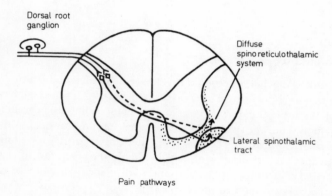

Pain pathways

Fig. 4.2 Spinal pathways for pain. (From Lance and McLeod, 1981, with permission of Butterworths, London.)

ipsilateral dorsal columns without synapsing. Tactile afferents pass through both ipsilateral dorsal columns and contralateral ventrolateral columns (Fig. 4.3).

The dorsal columns

The dorsal columns (i) transmit the sensation of light touch; (ii) are important in spatial discrimination of tactile stimuli (e.g. two-point discrimination); and (iii) transmit joint position and vibration sense,

Touch and proprioceptive pathways

Fig. 4.3 Spinal pathways for proprioception and touch. (From Lance and McLeod, 1981, with permission of Butterworths, London.)

although transmission of these modalities may not be exclusively a posterior column function.

The ventrolateral columns

The ventrolateral columns transmit (i) pain and temperature sensation; (ii) light touch sensation (the threshold for tactile sensation is raised after transection of the anterolateral columns); (iii) sensations of tickle and itch; (iv) sexual sensations; and (v) vibration sense. The ability to perceive vibration may be impaired or lost in lesions of the lateral columns.

The endogenous pain control system

The transmission of pain impulses from afferent fibres entering the dorsal horn to the second order neurones is inhibited by activity in large diameter low-threshold fibres and is also regulated by descending pathways from the brainstem (Fig. 4.4). The nucleus raphe magnus of the medulla controls pain transmission in the spinal cord through a descending serotoninergic pathway. The locus coeruleus and adjacent areas influence pain transmission through a noradrenergic pathway. The periaqueductal grey matter in the midbrain contains opiate receptors and enkephalins, and descending pathways from this region to the brainstem and spinal cord inhibit pain transmission.

Fig. 4.4 Endogenous pain control system. The periaqueductal grey matter (PAG) of the midbrain projects caudally through the nucleus raphe magnus (NRM) of the medulla to the spinal cord where 5-hydroxytryptamine (serotonin) is released as a neurotransmitter. A complementary noradrenergic pathway descends from the locus coeruleus (LC) through the dorsolateral fasciculus (DLF) to the spinal cord. First order neurons (FON) carrying pain impulses synapse in the dorsal horn with second order neurons (SON) that transmit impulses rostrally in the spinothalamic tract (STT). Transmission at this synapse is regulated by inhibitory interneurons (IN) which in turn are controlled by the descending pain control fibres in the DLF.

Modalities of sensation

Light touch

Clinically light touch is usually tested with cotton wool. Large myelinated fibres (A$\alpha\beta$) are excited by light touch, but not exclusively so since Aδ and C fibres are also excited by stroking the skin with cotton wool.

Fig. 4.5 Cerebral termination of sensory pathways. Specific afferent pathways are indicated as solid lines on the left of the diagram, fibres from the face synapsing in the posteroventromedial nucleus (VPM) of the thalamus on their way to the cortex, while fibres from the rest of the body synapse in the posteroventrolateral nucleus (VPL). Diffuse spinoreticulothalamic pain fibres are shown as interrupted lines on the right side of the diagram, synapsing in the midline thalamic nuclei, centrum medianum (CM) and lateral reticular nucleus (LR) before projecting widely to the cerebral cortex. (From Lance and McLeod, 1981, with permission of Butterworths, London.)

Human experiments indicate that tactile sensation may be induced by the excitation of only one or two large myelinated fibres.

Impulses excited in the periphery by light touch are conducted centrally in the spinal cord by way of the dorsal columns, through the medial lemniscal system to the opposite thalamus (posterolateral ventral nucleus) and thence to the cerebral cortex (Figs 4.3, 4.5). Tactile sensation is also conveyed in the ventrolateral columns in an ill-defined tract, the ventral spinothalamic tract (Fig. 4.3).

Joint position sense

Information concerning the orientation of the body in space and the spatial relations between its parts is derived from input from the visual apparatus, vestibular receptors and somatic sensory system. The somatic sensory component — kinaesthesia, or the sense of position and movement of joints — depends mainly upon receptor organs associated with joints that signal static position as well as changes in position. Recent evidence indicates that muscle spindles also play a role in the signalling of kinaesthesia.

Afferent fibres from joint receptors project through the dorsal columns and the lemniscal system to the sensory cortex (Figs 4.3, 4.5). Destruction of the dorsal columns results in impairment of position sense.

Vibration

The testing of vibration is merely a specialized way of testing tactile receptors and their pathways; there is probably no specific modality of vibration.

The peripheral pathway consists of large afferent fibres which innervate one or two Pacinian corpuscles. Pacinian corpuscles rapidly adapt and are very sensitive to vibration. The central pathway is by way of the dorsal columns to the lemniscal system, but spinocerebellar pathways also seem to play some part.

Pain

In any clinical consideration of pain, the psychological aspects and the patient's reaction to the sensation are of the utmost importance. However, the present discussion will be confined to anatomical and physiological aspects.

The adequate stimulus for pain threatens tissue damage, and in testing for painful sensation it is important that the patient recognizes the feeling of sharpness and not simply the feeling of contact or pressure.

There do not appear to be any specific receptors for pain in the skin or deep tissues. Impulses giving rise to painful sensation are initiated from free nerve endings.

It is well established in man as well as in experimental animals that the small myelinated Aδ fibres (which conduct impulses at velocities of 10–20 m/s) and the unmyelinated C fibres (which conduct at velocities of 1–2 m/s) are required to be stimulated before painful sensations are aroused. Stimulation of the C fibres gives rise to a most unpleasant quality of pain sensation and, because of the slower rate of conduction, the phenomenon of 'second pain' which is felt 1–2 s after the initial stab of pain. Although most pain impulses enter the spinal cord through the dorsal root, there is evidence that some traverse the ventral root so that pain may persist after dorsal rhizotomy. Impulses are transmitted in the spinal cord in the lateral spinothalamic tracts to the posterolateral ventral nucleus of the thalamus. Pathways probably then project to the sensory cortex so that impairment of pain sensation may sometimes follow localized injury to the sensory cortex in man.

A second pathway, the spinoreticulothalamic system (Fig. 4.2) is responsible for the transmission of diffuse poorly localized pain and travels to the reticular formation and midline thalamic nuclei (Fig. 4.5).

Itching

Itching is closely related to pain in its physiological mechanisms and its anatomical pathways.

Tickle

Tickle is probably a combination of tactile and painful sensations.

Temperature sense

Specific warm and cold endings exist. Both small myelinated and unmyelinated C fibres respond to thermal stimulation. The central pathways are closely related to those subserving painful sensation.

Higher centres

All sensory modalities, with the possible exception of pain, project from the thalamus to the sensory cortex in the post-central gyrus (Brodmann areas 3, 2, 1) (Figs 3.9, 4.5). Sensations are analysed in the sensory association areas of the parietal lobe (Brodmann areas 5, 7) (Fig. 12.1). Disturbances of these areas, which may be physiological as in drifting off to sleep, or pathological as in migraine or epilepsy, may cause illusions of body parts growing larger or smaller, or sensory hallucinations. Parietal lobe lesions may cause neglect of, or inattention to, a contralateral stimulus if two stimuli are presented simultaneously to both sides of the body (tactile inattention, see Chapter 12), or inability to recognize common objects (tactile agnosia). Two-point discrimination, position sense and stereognosis (recognition of the shape of objects) may be impaired if there is damage to the sensory cortex but will also be impaired by lesions of pathways at a lower level.

References

Lindblom U. and Ochoa J. (1986) Somatosensory function and dysfunction. In: *Diseases of the Nervous System*, pp. 283–98. Eds A. K. Asbury, G. M. McKhann and W. I. McDonald. W. B. Saunders, Philadelphia.

Maciewicz R. and Fields H.L. (1986) Pain pathways. In: *Diseases of the Nervous System*, pp. 930–40. Eds A. K. Asbury, G. M. McKhann and W. I. McDonald. W. B. Saunders, Philadelphia.

Sinclair D. (1981) *Mechanisms of Cutaneous Sensation*. Oxford University Press, Oxford.

5 Peripheral Neuropathy

The peripheral nervous system may be affected by injury or by disease processes. *Mononeuropathy* refers to a condition affecting a single nerve trunk, the most usual cause of which is trauma or entrapment. *Mononeuritis multiplex* is the term used to describe involvement by a disease process of several individual nerve trunks in an asymmetrical fashion. *Polyneuropathy* or *peripheral neuritis* indicates a widespread symmetrical process affecting the peripheral nervous system.

Structure of peripheral nerves

The peripheral nervous system consists of motor and sensory neurones and autonomic nerves. It includes the dorsal and ventral spinal roots, dorsal root and other sensory ganglia, sensory and motor terminals, spinal and cranial nerves and the peripheral autonomic nervous system (Fig. 5.1). Nerve trunks contain fascicles or bundles of individual nerve fibres separated by connective tissue (endoneurium) (Fig. 5.2). Each fascicle is surrounded by a fibrous connective tissue layer (perineurium); whole nerve trunks consist of a variable number of fascicles that are

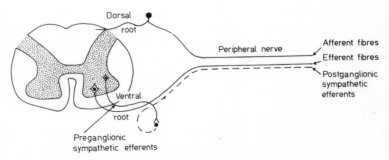

Fig. 5.1 Schematic representation of components of peripheral nerve trunks. (From Lance and McLeod, 1981, with permission of Butterworths, London.)

Fig. 5.2 Structure of peripheral nerve trunk and its blood supply. Regional arteries running longitudinally outside the nerve trunk supply nutrient arteries that penetrate the epineurium and form an anastomosis. Small arterioles perforate the epineurium of the fascicles and form an endoneurial capillary network. (Modified from P.J. Dyck, *Postgraduate Medicine*, 1967, **41**: 279–289).

contained within a loose connective tissue sheath (epineurium). Nerve trunks receive their blood supply from branches of regional arteries; small nutrient vessels penetrate the epineurium and form anastomoses within the nerve trunk.

Single nerve fibres within fascicles may be myelinated or un-myelinated. The motor axons are extensions of motor neurones in the anterior horns; the sensory axons are derived from dorsal root ganglion cells; and postganglionic sympathetic efferent fibres are unmyelinated and arise from ganglia in the thoracolumbar sympathetic chain (Chapter 7).

Myelinated fibres range in diameter from 2 to 22 μm; unmyelinated fibres diameters range from 0.2 to 3 μm. The satellite cell of the peripheral nervous system is the Schwann cell which is associated with both myelinated and unmyelinated fibres.

Myelinated fibres are characterized by their myelin sheaths which consist of alternating layers of protein and lipid and act as an insulating membrane around the axon. The myelin is interrupted at regular intervals by the nodes of Ranvier (Fig. 3.8). The segment of nerve between two successive nodes is an internode. Internodal length and myelin thickness are directly proportional to the external diameter of the nerve fibre. Myelin is the fusion of apposing layers of Schwann cell cytoplasmic membrane formed by the spiralling of the Schwann cell around the axon; myelin is thus not only formed by, but is actually a living part of, the Schwann cell. There is only one Schwann cell for each internode of the myelinated fibre, but by contrast there may be several unmyelinated fibres associated with a single Schwann cell.

Pathological reactions

Four major pathological processes may affect peripheral nerves (Fig. 5.3):

(a) Wallerian degeneration.
(b) Axonal degeneration.
(c) Segmental demyelination.
(d) Neuronopathy or primary nerve cell degeneration.

Wallerian degeneration

Wallerian degeneration is the process that follows mechanical injury such as transection or crush of nerve fibres, or it may follow ischaemic damage (e.g. vasculitis). Within a period of 4–5 days the axon and the myelin degenerate distal to the site of injury; the myelin forms linear arrays of ovoids and globules along the degenerating axon. The axon of the proximal segment then regenerates forming sprouts which grow distally, re-innervating the surviving distal neurilemmal tubes of

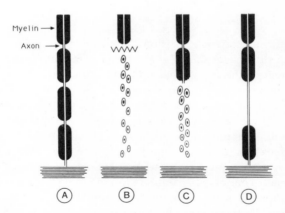

Fig. 5.3 Schematic representation of pathological changes in peripheral nerve fibres. (A) Normal myelinated fibre. (B) Wallerian degeneration following crush or section of nerve fibre. Axon and myelin degenerate. (C) Axonal degeneration of distal portion of nerve fibre in 'dying-back' neuropathy. Axon and myelin are both degenerating. (D) Segmental demyelination. Myelin has degenerated in one internode but axon remains intact.

Schwann cell basement membrane inside which the Schwann cells have divided and arranged themselves in line. The regenerating axons are then myelinated by the Schwann cells but the nerve fibres are of smaller diameter and have disproportionately short internodal lengths compared with the original fibres. Some regenerated axons never reach their distal connections.

Axonal degeneration

Axonal degeneration is the most common pathological change in peripheral neuropathies and is seen in most nutritional, metabolic and toxic causes of peripheral nerve disease. The pathological appearances in nerve biopsy specimens are similar to those of Wallerian degeneration. The usual mechanism is that disturbance of the metabolism of the cell body, or perikaryon, results in impairment of fast axonal transport and other functions so that the most distal parts of the axon, which may be as far removed as 1 m from the cell body, are first affected and die back from the periphery ('dying-back neuropathy'). Because the longest and usually largest diameter nerve fibres are first affected, distal muscle wasting and glove-and-stocking sensory loss are the usual clinical manifestations.

Segmental demyelination

Segmental demyelination is the term applied to the process of primary damage of the myelin sheath while the axon remains intact. In inflammatory neuropathies (e.g. Guillain-Barré syndrome) it is caused by a direct immune-mediated attack on the myelin or possibly on the Schwann cell. It may also result from presumed disturbances of Schwann cell metabolism in some hereditary neuropathies (e.g. Dejerine-Sottas disease) or toxic damage of the myelin sheath (experimental neuropathies produced with diphtheria, triethyl tin). When demyelination is severe there may be secondary axonal degeneration. Demyelination usually commences paranodally and often affects proximal parts of the peripheral nervous system (e.g. roots) to an equal or greater extent than the distal regions. When remyelination occurs, Schwann cells divide and form new internodes of irregular length with thin myelin sheaths. Repeated episodes of demyelination will result in the formation of concentric layers of Schwann cell cytoplasm and endoneurial elements around the axon which are described as 'onion bulb' formations.

Neuronopathies

In neuronopathies there is primary destruction of the nerve cell body. Examples of motor neuronopathies in which anterior horn cells are primarily affected are the spinal muscular atrophies, amyotrophic lateral sclerosis, and poliomyelitis. Sensory neuronopathies in which the dorsal root ganglion cell is primarily affected include Friedreich's ataxia and hereditary sensory neuropathies; there is distal degeneration of both peripheral sensory axons and the central processes ascending in the posterior columns and other spinal tracts. Since the cell bodies are destroyed in these disorders, there is no prospect of recovery.

Neurophysiology

In *Wallerian degeneration* nerve fibres continue to conduct impulses with normal or near normal conduction velocities until conduction ceases altogether 3–4 days following transection when the nerve fibres become totally inexcitable. Conduction is restored following regeneration but conduction velocities rarely attain their previous values.

In *axonal degeneration* conduction fails over the distal degenerating part of the axon in the same way as it does in Wallerian degeneration, but the intact proximal segments conduct with normal conduction velocities. Since clinical neurophysiological techniques measure conduction in the fastest conducting fibres and conduction velocities remain normal in individual fibres until conduction fails completely, there is only a mild reduction in velocities (usually less than 20–30%) which is due to the failure of conduction in large fibres. The measured conduction velocity is in the normally conducting unaffected smaller diameter fibres.

In *segmental demyelination* there are two major physiological consequences of demyelination, conduction block and slowing of conduction. Conduction block is the complete failure of nerve fibres to transmit electrical impulses across a demyelinated segment; it may be seen following acute nerve compression (e.g. after prolonged application of a tourniquet or pneumatic cuff) and in the inflammatory neuropathies (Guillain-Barré syndrome and chronic inflammatory demyelinating neuropathy). Slowing of conduction is usually quite marked across demyelinated or remyelinating segments of nerve. In normal myelinated fibres the impulses conduct rapidly from node to node by saltatory conduction, but in demyelinated nerve fibres either conduction becomes continuous across the demyelinated segments as it is in unmyelinated fibres, or conduction time between nodes is delayed. Other abnormalities of conduction that occur in demyelinated fibres are impairment of the ability to transmit faithfully rapid trains of impulses, increased irritability to mechanical stimulation, generation of spontaneous impulses from the demyelinated zones and an increased susceptibility to change in temperature.

Electromyography

Electromyography (EMG) is the recording of electrical activity from muscles through a needle electrode. The action potentials are displayed on a cathode ray oscilloscope and may be heard through a loud speaker. Normally there is no electrical activity recorded at rest, but in nerve injuries and diseases that damage axons spontaneous electrical activity (*spontaneous fibrillation*) arising from denervated muscle fibres may be detected 7–10 days after the injury (Fig. 3.7). In a complete nerve lesion no motor unit activity will be recorded following attempted voluntary effort or electrical stimulation of the nerve. In a partial injury the number of motor units will be reduced (see Fig. 3.6). If re-innervation of muscles has occurred, giant motor unit action potentials may be recorded because sprouting axons make contact with muscle fibres from other motor units, thus extending their original territory.

Nerve conduction studies

Nerve conduction studies are normally carried out on patients with suspected peripheral nerve disease. They are useful in confirming the presence of a generalized peripheral neuropathy and may indicate the nature of the underlying pathology. In mononeuropathies they may indicate the site of entrapment or of focal pathology.

With a needle in a muscle or a surface eletrode over the muscle belly, the action potential may be recorded following electrical stimulation of the motor nerve through surface electrodes on the skin. After suitable amplification and display on an oscilloscope the delay or latency between the time of stimulus and the onset of muscle action potential may be measured. If the nerve is stimulated at two separate points the conduction velocity of the volley in the segment of the nerve between the two points can be calculated; this is a measure of conduction in the fastest conducting fibres in the nerves (Fig. 5.4). In normal adults, the velocity in the fastest conducting motor fibres of the median and ulnar nerves in the forearm is approximately 50–65 m/s and is somewhat less, about 40–50 m/s, in the nerves of the lower limbs.

Conduction velocities are a little greater in proximal than in distal segments of the nerves. In full-term newborn infants the motor conduction velocity is approximately one-half that of the adult value and increases with age to approach adult values at about 3–5 years. Since

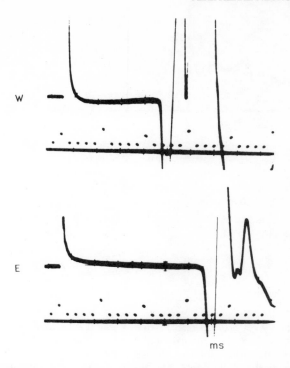

Fig. 5.4 Muscle action potentials recorded with a concentric needle electrode from abductor pollicis brevis muscle on stimulating the median nerve at the wrist (W) and elbow (E) in a patient with a carpal tunnel syndrome. The latency of response from wrist to muscle is prolonged (11.2 ms) beyond the normal value (<5 ms). Latency from elbow to muscle is 16.3 ms. Conduction time from elbow to wrist is $16.2 - 11.2 = 5.0$ ms. Conduction distance between stimulating electrodes = 23 cm. Motor conduction velocity in forearm is $230/5 = 66$ ms. (From Lance and McLeod, 1981, with permission of Butterworths, London.)

conduction velocities decrease by approximately 2 m/s per °C, over the range 36–26°C, it is important to maintain careful control of limb temperature. Conduction is delayed through regions of localized injury or disease, e.g. the median nerve at the wrist in carpal tunnel syndrome.

Sensory action potentials may be recorded through surface electrodes from the median and ulnar nerves at the wrist by electrically stimulating the digital nerves in the index and little fingers respectively through ring electrodes (Fig. 5.5). Sensory conduction can also be recorded in radial, sural and saphenous nerves. Mixed (motor and sen-

Fig. 5.5 Sensory action potential recorded from the median nerve at the wrist with surface electrodes on the skin (R) following electrical stimulation of digital nerves at the index finger through ring electrodes (S). Time marker 1 ms intervals. (From Lance and McLeod, 1981, with permission of Butterworths, London.)

sory) nerve action potentials may be recorded from nerve trunks such as those of the median, ulnar and common peroneal nerves. Abnormalities of latency, amplitude and conduction velocity of sensory and mixed nerve action potentials are usually a more sensitive index of the presence of a neuropathy than changes in the motor conduction velocities.

In axonal degeneration the conduction velocity of the fastest fibres will be only slightly reduced since the fibres that are undamaged by the disease process conduct with normal conduction velocities and those that are degenerating do not conduct at all. The amplitude of the compound action potential will be smaller because fewer motor units are activated by the stimulus. In segmental demyelination, conduction velocities may be reduced to less than 60% of their normal values. Conduction block is also a feature of acute demyelination; it is assessed by attenuation of the compound action potential when the stimulus is moved from a distal to a proximal site. Temporal dispersion of the action potential is seen in demyelination and remyelination. The distal latency may be disproportionately prolonged in demyelinating neuropathies.

The H-reflex (named after Hoffman who described it) is a monosynaptic reflex recorded from a muscle following electrical stimulation at a low intensity of stimulus of large afferent fibres originating from that muscle. It is thus comparable to the tendon jerk, although the transducer action of the muscle spindle is by-passed by direct electrical stimulation of the muscle afferents. It is most conveniently recorded from calf muscles and is decreased or absent in most peripheral neuropathies.

The F-wave is recorded in a similar manner to the H-reflex and is caused by backfiring of motor neurones in response to antidromic electrical stimulation of motor fibres. The latency of the F-wave is a measure of the time of conduction in motor fibres from the site of stimulation to the motor neurone and then back to the recording site. It is a useful measure of conduction in proximal segments of nerve roots.

Diseases of the peripheral nervous system

The peripheral nervous system may be affected by localized injury to peripheral nerve trunks or roots, vascular occlusions in major nerve trunks (e.g. in polyarteritis or diabetes), or generalized disease processes affecting the function of peripheral nerves. Some of the causes of peripheral neuropathy are listed below. The most common are diabetes, alcohol, nutritional deficiencies, and, in many countries, leprosy.

Genetically determined neuropathies

Charcot-Marie-Tooth disease (peroneal muscular atrophy) has an autosomal dominant inheritance and is the most common genetically determined neuropathy. Symptoms usually begin at 10–30 years of age. The earliest signs are distal wasting of the lower limbs with foot-drop. The intrinsic hand muscles become affected later and mild distal sensory loss is usually apparent. Reflexes in the lower limbs are depressed or absent. The foot has a characteristic appearance with a high arch and retracted toes (pes cavus). The condition progresses very slowly over many years. Two major types are recognized:
(a) Heredity motor and sensory neuropathy type I (HMSN type I) or the hypertrophic type, in which the peripheral nerves are thickened and segmental demyelination is the underlying pathology.
(b) HMSN type II, the neuronal type, in which there is axonal degeneration without hypertrophic changes.

Other less common hereditary peripheral neuropathies include the hereditary sensory neuropathies in which mutilating deformities develop in the hands and feet, and a severe hypertrophic neuropathy, Dejerine-Sottas disease, which usually presents in childhood. The peripheral nerves may be affected in a number of other hereditary diseases that also affect the central nervous system (e.g. Friedreich's ataxia, metachromatic leukodystrophy).

Drugs and other toxins

Heavy metals (arsenic, lead, mercury, thallium, gold), industrial agents (acrylamide, hexacarbons, triorthocresyl phosphate), and drugs (isoniazid, ethambutol, nitrofurantoin, vincristine, phenytoin, thalidomide, lithium carbonate, perhexiline, chloroquin, disulfiram) may cause a peripheral neuropathy. Generalized peripheral neuropathy or mononeuritis multiplex may sometimes follow as an allergic or immune response to vaccinations and injections of foreign proteins.

Metabolic and endocrine

Diabetes is a common cause of peripheral neuropathy, usually symmetrical and predominantly sensory. When there is severe sensory impairment, perforating ulcers of the feet and neuropathic joints (Charcot joints) may occur with associated sensory ataxia. Symptoms of autonomic dysfunction are common. *Diabetic amyotrophy* is a painful asymmetrical proximal neuropathy affecting predominantly the quadriceps, hamstring and gluteal muscles of the lower limbs. Isolated peripheral nerve lesions particularly the carpal tunnel syndrome and ulnar nerve lesions at the elbow are also common.

Uraemia, porphyria, acromegaly, hypothyroidism and recurrent attacks of hypoglycaemia due to islet cell tumours of the pancreas may also be associated with peripheral neuropathies.

Vitamin deficiencies

Vitamin B_{12} deficiency, whether associated with pernicious anaemia or malabsorption syndromes, results in a predominantly sensory neuropathy that may be accompanied by subacute combined degeneration of the spinal cord (p. 106). Vitamin B_1 (thiamine) deficiency is seen particularly in chronic alcoholism and severe nutritional disturbances and causes a painful, predominantly sensory neuropathy.

Alcohol is one of the commonest causes of peripheral neuropathy in urban populations. Common symptoms are pains in the calves, burning feet and distal weakness. Distal muscle wasting, absent knee and ankle jerks and distal sensory impairment with tender calves are the usual physical findings. It is caused by Vitamin B deficiency rather than by the direct effects of alcohol.

Malignancies

Clinical peripheral neuropathy occurs as a remote (paraneoplastic) manifestation in about 5% of patients with carcinoma and lymphoma. A predominantly sensory ganglionopathy occurs in association with small-cell carcinoma of the lung. Paraproteinaemias and dysproteinaemias (e.g. multiple myeloma, macroglobulinaemia) are often associated with peripheral neuropathy.

Connective tissue diseases

Rheumatoid arthritis may be accompanied by a symmetrical sensory or sensorimotor neuropathy. Mononeuritis multiplex caused by arteritis, and entrapment neuropathies are also well recognized complications of rheumatoid disease.

Polyarteritis nodosa classically causes a mononeuritis multiplex which may also be seen in systemic lupus erythematosus (SLE) and sarcoidosis.

Infections

Leprosy is the most common cause of peripheral neuropathy on a worldwide basis. *Mycobacterium leprae* invades the Schwann cell.

Inflammatory neuropathies

Guillain-Barré syndrome (acute inflammatory polyneuritis) has a rapid onset and is potentially fatal. The common initial symptoms of paraesthesiae or pain in the lower limbs are followed by weakness; because nerve roots are also involved in the inflammatory process, proximal muscles may be affected to the same or even a greater extent than the distal muscle groups. Facial and bulbar paralysis are common and there may be weakness of the extraocular muscles. Reflexes are usually depressed or absent and there is a variable degree of sensory loss. Within 3–4 weeks this predominantly motor neuropathy progresses to a maximum disability often with complete quadriparesis and respiratory paralysis. About 80% of patients recover without any significant disability, but about 5% of cases relapse. Typically the protein level in cerebrospinal fluid is elevated and the cell count is not increased. It is likely that the pathogenesis of the disorder is a cell-mediated immune response directed at myelin in peripheral nerve and spinal roots, which may be provoked by certain viral infections since these precede the onset of the condition in about 60% of cases. *Chronic inflammatory neuropathy* has a slower onset and may run a relapsing and remitting course.

Clinical features of peripheral neuropathy

Most chronic polyneuropathies are symmetrical, predominantly distal and have a mixture of motor and sensory manifestations. Motor symptoms are those of weakness of distal muscles; patients find difficulty in climbing stairs and difficulty in unfastening buttons or performing fine movements. Muscle wasting, foot-drop and wrist-drop are common. Sensory disturbances include numbness, tingling, pins and needles in the hands and feet, burning sensations, pain in the extremities, sensations of walking on cotton wool and band-like constrictions around the wrists or ankles, unsteadiness on the feet or stumbling. Autonomic dysfunction may be manifested as a dryness or excessive sweating of the extremities, postural hypotension, diarrhoea and constipation.

The signs of peripheral neuropathy are usually those of distal muscle wasting and weakness and sensory impairment, often in a glove-and-stocking type of distribution. Two-point discrimination is the most sensitive test of mild degrees of sensory impairment. Reflexes are usually depressed or absent, but in mild cases the abnormalities may be confined to the ankle jerks since their pathway is longer than that of other reflexes.

The clinical features of sensory impairment, distal muscle wasting and weakness and early loss of reflexes, distinguish peripheral neuropathies from myopathies (see pp. 76–77).

Onset and course

Most neuropathies have a gradual onset and slow progression. Acute onset of neuropathy is seen only in a limited number of conditions which include the Guillain-Barré syndrome, porphyria, diphtheria, acute toxic neuropathies, and neuropathies that follow vaccinations and injections.

Pattern of distribution

Most neuropathies have a symmetrical distribution and affect the lower limbs to a greater extent than the upper limbs. Some neuropathies have an asymmetrical presentation and these include the acute and chronic inflammatory neuropathies and those caused by disease of small blood vessels. Mononeuritis multiplex suggests a vascular cause (polyarteritis, rheumatoid arthritis, small vessel disease in diabetes) but other aetiological factors such as sarcoidosis, leprosy and autoimmune reactions to injections and vaccinations must be considered.

Brachial neuritis (neuralgic amyotrophy) is a condition characterized by the rapid onset of pain, weakness and wasting of the muscles of one shoulder and upper arm, although it is sometimes bilateral. Its onset may be related to an infection or injection, but in most cases there are no recognized precipitating factors.

Most neuropathies characteristically have a distal distribution but proximal weakness may be a feature of porphyria, acute and chronic demyelinating neuropathies and Dejerine-Sottas disease. Lower limbs are usually affected earlier and to a greater extent than the upper limbs; exceptions to the rule are acute and chronic demyelinating neuropathies, porphyria and lead poisoning.

Predominantly motor or sensory neuropathies

Some peripheral neuropathies affect either mainly motor or mainly sensory fibres (Table 5.1), although most have manifestations of both. When large sensory fibres are predominantly affected (e.g. Friedreich's ataxia) light touch, vibration and position sense are characteristically impaired with sparing of pain and temperature sensations and loss of reflexes. In some other neuropathies (e.g. amyloidosis, diabetes) the small fibres are selectively involved causing autonomic dysfunction and burning pain associated with loss of pain and temperature sense whereas tactile sensation is relatively spared.

Nerve injuries

In nerve injuries three main disorders of function are recognized.

Neuropraxia

Neuropraxia is transient loss of function of a nerve following compression or mild trauma; spontaneous recovery of function occurs within

Table 5.1   Clinical types of peripheral neuropathy

Acute onset
    Guillain-Barré syndrome
    Porphyria
    Toxic
    Serum sickness (post-vaccinial)
    Malignancy
Predominantly motor
    Guillain-Barré syndrome
    Porphyria
    Diphtheria
    Lead
    Charcot-Marie-Tooth disease
Predominantly sensory
    Leprosy
    Diabetes
    Vitamin B_{12} or thiamine deficiency
    Malignancy
    Hereditary sensory neuropathy
    Amyloid disease
    Uraemia
Painful neuropathies
    Alcohol, nutritional deficiencies
    Diabetes
    Hereditary sensory neuropathy
    Arsenic
    Cryoglobulinaemia

days or weeks. The underlying pathology is local demyelination; temporary localized block in conduction of the nerve impulse can be demonstrated at the affected site. The axon of the nerve remains intact.

Axonotmesis

Axonotmesis results from crush injuries that cause degeneration of the axon and its myelin sheath (Wallerian degeneration). The neurilemmal sheaths, consisting of tubes of basement membranes, are preserved and are re-innervated by the regenerating axons.

Neurotmesis

This is the condition in which the whole nerve trunk is severed and continuity of the neurilemmal sheath is lost. The distal nerve trunk cannot be re-innervated effectively unless surgical repair is undertaken to approximate, as accurately as possible, the proximal and distal ends of the nerve trunk.

Entrapment and compression neuropathies

Isolated nerve trunks are frequently affected by entrapment or compression in anatomical compartments. The most common example is compression of the median nerve beneath the flexor retinaculum at the wrist causing the *carpal tunnel syndrome*. The condition is more common in women and may be bilateral. Narrowing of the carpal tunnel occurs in obesity, myxoedema, acromegaly, fluid retention caused by use of oral contraceptive pills or pregnancy, rheumatoid arthritis or wrist trauma. The symptoms are numbness and tingling in the thumb and fingers supplied by the median nerve (index, middle and radial half of the ring finger) mainly at night and if the nerve has been entrapped for long periods of time there are signs of sensory loss over the median nerve distribution of the hand and wasting of the thenar muscles.

Other well recognized entrapment syndromes are compression of the ulnar nerve at the elbow causing paraesthesiae and sensory loss in the little and ulnar half of the ring finger, and wasting and weakness of the interossei; compression of the peroneal nerve at the neck of the fibula resulting in foot-drop and numbness over the dorsum of the foot and lateral aspect of the leg; compression of the lateral cutaneous nerve of the thigh, which occurs particularly in people who are overweight and causes numbness and tingling over the outer aspect of the thigh (meralgia paraesthetica); and radial nerve lesions at the lower end of the spiral groove of the humerus causing wrist-drop. Predisposing factors to entrapment neuropathies are repetitive trauma, diabetes, alcoholism and other causes of peripheral nerve disease. Surgical decompression of the nerve may be necessary.

Investigations

The basic investigations that should be performed on all patients with peripheral neuropathy of unknown cause include urinalysis, full blood count, measurement of erythrocyte sedimentation rate, fasting blood sugar, serum electrolytes, serum creatinine, serum proteins and immunoelectrophoresis, liver function tests and serum Vitamin B_{12} levels. Serum lipoproteins, urinary porphyrins, heavy metals, amino acids, and faecal fats, should be studied in appropriate cases. Examination of the cerebrospinal fluid may be helpful in some cases (e.g. Guillain-Barré syndrome). Other investigations to exclude malignancy may include chest X-ray and other appropriate radiological and endoscopic investigations.

Treatment

Acute neuropathies

In the Guillain-Barré syndrome and other peripheral neuropathies with acute involvement of respiratory muscles, spirometry should be performed every 2–4 h in the initial stages because tracheal intubation or tracheostomy and artificial ventilation may be necessary. Careful nursing is very important and particular attention should be paid to the care of the skin, bladder, bowels, mouth, pharynx and trachea. Lung and urinary tract infections require prompt treatment. Intravenous or intragastric feeding may be necessary. Physiotherapy should begin immediately and splints to prevent foot- and wrist-drop may be required. Plasmapheresis hastens recovery and improves prognosis if commenced within days of onset of Guillain-Barré syndrome. Corticosteroids do not have a beneficial effect.

Chronic neuropathies

Specific treatment for the underlying cause should be given when indicated. Corticosteroids, immunosuppressive therapy and plasmapheresis may be helpful in patients with chronic inflammatory neuropathy. Physiotherapy is an important part of treatment. In severe cases splints, calipers and other walking aids will be necessary and occasionally surgical corrective procedures will be required. A programme of rehabilitation should be commenced.

References

Aids to the Examination of the Peripheral Nervous System (1986) Baillière Tindall.

Asbury A.K. and Gilliatt R.W. (eds) (1984) *Peripheral Nerve Disorders*. Butterworths, London.

Dyck P.K., Thomas P.K., Lambert E.H. and Bunge R. (eds) (1984) *Peripheral Neuropathy*. W.B. Saunders, Philadelphia.

Schaumburg H.H., Spencer P.S. and Thomas P.K. (1983) *Disorders of the Peripheral Nervous System*. F.A. Davis, Philadelphia.

Sumner A.J. (ed) (1980) *The Physiology of Peripheral Nerve Disease*. W.B. Saunders, Philadelphia.

6 Diseases of Muscle and the Neuromuscular Junction

Structure of muscle

Muscles are composed of many parallel fibres, each of which is a large multinucleated cell enclosed by a sarcolemmal membrane. The sarcoplasm within the cell contains myofibrils which constitute the contractile machinery of the muscle as well as mitochondria that contain oxidative enzymes and other cellular constituents. Each myofibril is about 1 μm in diameter and is composed of precisely aligned thick (myosin) and thin (actin) filaments which alternate to form a repetitive band pattern, giving rise to the cross-striated appearance of muscle fibres that is apparent on light and electron microscopy (Fig. 6.1). The dark A band contains overlapping thick and thin filaments and the light I band contains only the thin actin filaments. At the centre of the A band is a dark H band composed only of myosin with the M line at its centre. The dense Z line at the centre of the I band represents the attachment of the actin fibres and is composed of desmin, alpha actinin and amorphin. The sarcomere is the unit between two successive Z lines and is about 2–3 μm in length.

Fig. 6.1 Schematic representation of a myofibril. Thick myosin (thick band) filaments overlap thin actin (thin band) filaments. A sarcomere lies between two Z bands. A, I, H and M refer to bands seen on electron microscopy.

The myofibrils are closely embraced by the sarcoplasmic reticulum in which calcium is stored. The T system consists of tubules which run transversely, usually at the junction of the A and I bands. The T tubules arise as an invagination of the sarcolemmal membrane and are in direct continuity with the extracellular fluid.

When the muscle end-plate is depolarized, an action potential is propagated down the muscle fibre and along the T system leading to the release of calcium ions from the sarcoplasmic reticulum. The released calcium is bound by troponin, a protein associated with actin in the thin filament. When a muscle is at rest troponin and tropomyosin are linked and prevent actin from binding to myosin. The binding of calcium to troponin breaks the linkage resulting in the interaction between actin and myosin that causes muscle contraction. The energy for the process is obtained from the breakdown of ATP. Muscle fibre relaxation results from active pumping back of calcium ions into the sarcoplasmic reticulum.

Muscle fibres may be classified according to their speed of contraction. Slowly contracting fibres are rich in mitochondria and derive their energy from oxidative metabolism. Fast contracting fibres are rich in glycogen and derive their energy mainly through the glycolytic pathway. Histochemical staining with ATPase, succinic dehydrogenase, and other stains, will differentiate the type 1 (slow contracting aerobic metabolism) from the type 2 (fast conducting anaerobic metabolism) fibres. Histochemistry of muscle biopsies is very helpful in the diagnosis of muscle diseases.

Diseases of muscles

Diseases in which the muscle fibres are primarily affected are known as *myopathies*. They may be classified according to whether they are genetically determined or acquired. Genetically determined myopathies are known as muscular dystrophies. Myopathies must be distinguished from the neurogenic atrophies in which muscle wasting is secondary to disease of the anterior horn cells or peripheral nerves. In myopathies degenerative and metabolic changes occur primarily in the muscle fibres. In some conditions, there are distinctive morphological features.

Clinical features of muscle diseases

The onset is usually insidious. Proximal muscle groups are usually affected first and patients may notice difficulty in walking, rising from a chair, climbing stairs, hanging clothes on a line or combing the hair.

Facial weakness may be apparent in smiling and whistling, and weakness of bulbar muscles may be manifested by difficulty in chewing and swallowing. Pain is usually not a feature but may be present on exertion in McArdle's disease and polymyositis. A careful family history should always be taken in case there is a genetically determined disorder and the patient should be asked specifically whether there is any parental consanguinity. The distribution of weakness is variable and forms the basis for classification of muscular dystrophies. Usually proximal muscles are affected to a greater extent than distal muscles. Muscle tone and deep tendon reflexes are diminished in proportion to muscle weakness.

Clinical features that distinguish muscle diseases from peripheral neuropathies are their proximal distribution of weakness and wasting, the absence of sensory abnormalities and the relative preservation of reflexes.

Classification of muscle diseases

Genetically determined myopathies

Progressive muscular dystrophies
(a) *Duchenne muscular dystrophy*   This is the commonest form of progressive muscular dystrophy. It affects 13–33/100 000 live-born males and about 0.2–0.3% of the population. It is a sex-linked recessive disorder and, with rare exceptions, affects only males. Females are carriers of the disease. Onset occurs in the first decade of life and progresses to death from respiratory or cardiac failure usually in the second or third decade. Weakness usually begins in the proximal muscles of the lower limbs but soon spreads to involve the anterior tibial group of muscles, trunk muscles and proximal muscles of the upper limbs. The calf muscles are unusually prominent, initially due to muscle hypertrophy but later to fatty infiltration of degenerated muscles (pseudohypertrophy). The heart is usually affected and intellectual retardation is common. The serum creatine kinase (CK) levels are very high in affected children and are also elevated in carriers. Early detection of carriers is important for genetic counselling. The gene can now be localized with considerable accuracy on the X chromosome. A benign form (Becker type) is recognized.
(b) *Facioscapulohumeral muscular dystrophy*   This is autosomal dominant and has a later age of onset and slower progression than Duchenne muscular dystrophy. The muscles most affected are biceps, triceps, and

muscles of the shoulder girdle. Scapula winging is prominent. Facial muscles are also involved early but pelvic muscles are affected later in the course of the disease.

(c) *Limb girdle muscular dystrophy*   This is probably a heterogeneous group of conditions in which the shoulder and pelvic muscles are predominantly involved but facial muscles are spared. Most cases are sporadic or have an autosomal recessive inheritance.

(d) *Scapuloperoneal muscular dystrophy*   Shoulder girdle muscles and muscles of the anterolateral compartment of the leg are primarily affected. The condition may be X-linked or autosomal dominant.

(e) *Ocular myopathy (progressive external ophthalmoplegia)*   Ocular myopathies are characterized by progressive external ophthalmoplegia, ptosis and often facial weakness. They are a heterogeneous group of disorders, the most common of which is mitochondrial myopathy.

Myotonic dystrophies

These are genetically determined muscle disorders which are characterized by the presence of myotonia. *Myotonia* is the failure of the voluntary muscles to relax immediately after contraction and clinically it may be demonstrated by a slowness of relaxation of the hand grip or a prolonged dimpling of the muscle after being struck sharply with a percussion hammer (percussion myotonia). Electromyographically, myotonia is distinguished by prolonged spontaneous discharges from the resting muscle that commence at high frequency and then wane in both frequency and amplitude (Fig. 6.2). The myotonia is a manifestation of increased muscle cell membrane excitability due to reduced chloride conductance. Two main types are recognized — dystrophia myotonica and myotonia congenita.

(a) *Dystrophia myotonica* is a relatively common form of muscular dystrophy affecting about 5/100 000 of the population. Inheritance is autosomal dominant and the gene has been localized on chromosome 19. The onset is insidious usually between the ages of 20 and 50 years but it may be present in childhood or at birth. There is progressive wasting and weakness of distal as well as proximal muscles, ptosis, weakness of facial muscles, weakness and wasting of sternomastoids, cataracts, gonadal atrophy, frontal baldness, cardiomyopathy and abnormalities of insulin secretion.

(b) *Myotonia congenita (Thomsen's disease)*   There are both autosomal dominant and recessive varieties of this disease. The onset is usually in early life with myotonia and muscle stiffness which normally improves with exercise, but when it is severe attempts to run or walk may cause the patient to fall. The muscles are hypertrophied and strong, in contrast to those in patients with dystrophic myotonia.

├── 0·5 s ──┤

Fig. 6.2 Continuous electromyographic recording of myotonic discharge from muscle of a patient with dystrophia myotonica. Note that the amplitude of the action potential becomes progressively smaller and frequency of the discharge becomes progressively reduced with time. (From Lance and McLeod, 1981, with permission of Butterworths, London.)

Familial periodic paralyses

Recurrent attacks of weakness lasting several hours may be related to changes in the serum potassium level. The most common form is *hypokalaemic periodic paralysis* which has an autosomal dominant inheritance. During the attacks, which may be precipitated by rest after exercise or by heavy carbohydrate intake, there is a low level of serum potassium due to an intracellular shift of potassium and other ions. One particular form of hypokalaemic periodic paralysis is associated with thyrotoxicosis. *Hyperkalaemic periodic paralysis*, which is also transmitted by an autosomal dominant gene, is associated with raised serum potassium during attacks. In this type myotonia may be a feature. In a third type, *normokalaemic periodic paralysis*, potassium levels remain normal.

Mitochondrial myopathy

Mitochondrial myopathies are a group of disorders in which mitochondrial abnormalities are seen on muscle biopsy. The usual clinical manifestations are muscle weakness with fatiguability and progressive external ophthalmoplegia. Specific mitochondrial enzyme deficiencies have been demonstrated in some cases. They may be associated with evidence of degeneration of other systems, e.g. cerebellar ataxia, myoclonus, strokes.

Congenital myopathies

There is a large number of genetically determined myopathies of unknown aetiology which are characterized by their muscle biopsy appearances, e.g. central core disease, nemaline myopathy, centronuclear myopathy.

Other genetically determined metabolic disorders

Some muscle disorders are associated with abnormalities of glycogen metabolism. The best known is McArdle's syndrome in which there is a deficiency of muscle phosphorylase. The symptoms are fatigue, cramps on exertion and contracture of the muscles if exercise continues. In a similar disorder an inherited absence of fructokinase has been identified.

Myopathies may also be associated with inherited disorders of muscle lipid metabolism, e.g. carnitine deficiency.

Acquired myopathies

Myopathies, usually presenting with proximal muscle weakness, may be secondary to a number of different causes.

Endocrine Thyrotoxicosis, myxoedema, Cushing's disease, hyperparathyroidism, osteomalacia, acromegaly, steroid administration.

Toxic Alcohol, malignancy, drugs (e.g. corticosteroids, chloroquine).

Metabolic disturbances Potassium loss from vomiting, diarrhoea or urinary excretion may cause profound generalized weakness or even complete paralysis. Hypokalaemia may reach dangerous levels in: the recovery phase of diabetic coma; potassium-losing nephritis; aldosteronism; or long continued use of diuretic agents, adrenocorticosteroids or carbenoxolone sodium.

Polymyositis Polymyositis is an inflammatory reaction of muscle which most likely has an auto-immune basis. Patients usually present with muscle weakness, affecting predominantly proximal muscles, and in some cases this may be associated with muscle pain. The most common form is simple polymyositis in which no underlying cause is demonstrated, but it may also be associated with connective tissue diseases (e.g. systemic lupus erythematosus, progressive systemic sclerosis, rheumatoid arthritis), malignancy, and dermatomyositis (in which there is an accompanying skin rash).

Diseases of the neuromuscular junction

The nerve terminals of motor fibres lie in grooves, or gutters, in the muscle end-plates. The cell membranes of the nerve and muscles are separated by a space of about 50 nm (Fig. 6.3). At rest acetylcholine (ACh) is released spontaneously from synaptic vesicles in the nerve endings; it diffuses rapidly across the space to bind to acetylcholine receptors (AChR), partially depolarizing the muscle membrane and giving rise to miniature end-plate potentials (mepps) which may be recorded with an intracellular electrode in the end-plate zone. The mepps have a frequency of about 1 Hz and an amplitude of about 0.5–1.0 mV. Each mepp represents the release of a single packet or quantum of ACh (about 10 000 molecules) from a synaptic vesicle. When a nerve impulse arrives at the nerve terminal there is an enormous increase in the number of quanta of ACh released; as many as 250–500 may be liberated by each nerve impulse. Depolarization of the muscle membrane which follows results in the production of an end-plate potential (about 30–40 mV in amplitude) and the initiation of the muscle action potential. ACh is broken down by cholinesterase and subsequently resynthesized in the axon.

Abnormalities of neuromuscular transmission occur in myasthenia gravis and in the myasthenic syndrome associated with malignancy.

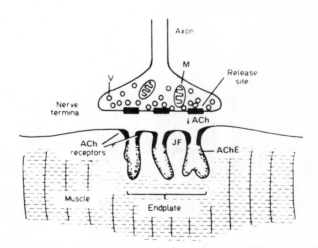

Fig. 6.3 Neuromuscular junction. V. vesicles; M, mitochondria; ACh, acetyl choline; JF, junctional folds; AChE, acetylcholine esterase (Modified from Drachman, 1978, *The New England Journal of Medicine* **298**, 136, with permission of the Editor.)

Myasthenia gravis

Clinical features

Patients with myasthenia gravis complain of rapid fatigue after muscular effort. Weakness is usually more pronounced at the end of the day and improved by rest. It may be confined to restricted muscle groups, especially the ocular muscles (ocular myasthenia); or it may become generalized. In severe cases respiratory muscles are involved. Patients often complain of double vision, drooping of the eyelids, alteration in speech, and difficulty in chewing and swallowing, as well as a weakness in the limbs. A snarling smile is characteristic of the myasthenic patient.

Thymic hyperplasia is present in the majority of patients with onset under the age of 40 years, and a thymoma is present in about 10% of all patients with myasthenia gravis. A computerized tomographic (CT) scan may reveal the thymic enlargement in the anterior mediastinum. The diagnosis may be confirmed by diagnostic procedures, the most important of which is the detection of anti-ACh receptor (anti-AChR) antibodies which are present in about 80–90% of cases. Repetitive electrical stimulation of a motor nerve at rates of 1–30 Hz causes a rapid and marked decline in the amplitude of the compound muscle action potential in myasthenia gravis patients in contrast to normals (Fig. 6.4). Intravenous injection of an anticholinesterase drug, edrophonium hydrochloride (Tensilon), (2 mg test dose followed by 8 mg) improves muscle strength for a period of 2–5 min. Single fibre electromyography

3 Hz

2 mV

Fig. 6.4 Myasthenic response to repetitive electrical stimulation of a nerve. Successive muscle action potentials were recorded with surface electrodes over abductor digiti minimi muscle on stimulating an ulnar nerve at a rate of 3 Hz. Note rapid decline in amplitude of muscle action potential. (From Lance and McLeod, 1981, with permission of Butterworths, London.)

allows impairment of neuromuscular transmission to be recorded electrophysiologically as a variable latency of different components of the motor unit ('jitter') and is useful in some cases where the diagnosis is in doubt.

Babies born to mothers with myasthenia gravis may have transient weakness due to the transplacental passage of maternal anti-AChR antibodies (*neonatal myasthenia*).

Pathogenesis

Anti-AChR antibody is an IgG antibody released mainly by thymic cells. These circulating antibodies become attached to, and inactivate, the muscle end-plate receptors, reducing the number of functioning endplates so that mepps are reduced in amplitude although normal in frequency.

Myasthenia gravis is known to have an auto-immune basis because of: the presence of anti-AChR antibodies, associated abnormalities of the thymus gland, the co-existence of auto-immune phenomena, and an association of certain HLA antigens (HLA-B8 and DW3) with onset under the age of 40 years. The thymus gland plays an important part in the pathogenesis of the condition; B lymphocytes and plasma cells in the gland release anti-AChR antibody, and there is frequently a favourable response to thymectomy.

Treatment

Anticholinesterase drugs are the main basis of the treatment. Neostigmine (Prostigmine), 15 mg or more every 3 h, or pyridostigmine (Mestinon), 60 mg or more every 4 h, is the usual therapy.

Thymectomy should be considered particularly in patients with onset less than 40 years of age, since it improves the long-term prognosis. It is not indicated in ocular myasthenia. Thymectomy is essential when a thymoma is present, and should be preceded or followed by radiotherapy. Immunosuppression with cortiocosteroids and azathioprine may be indicated particularly in patients who do not respond to anticholinesterase drugs.

Plasmapheresis may produce a dramatic but relatively short-lived response. It is used in patients with acute relapses of the disease who are not responding to other forms of therapy.

Myasthenia may sometimes be induced by penicillamine. Some antibiotics, including neomycin, kanamycin, streptomycin, bacitracin, colistin, ampicillin, and amoxicillin, interfere with neuromuscular transmission and their use should be avoided.

Myasthenic syndrome

A myasthenic syndrome is present in about 3% of patients with small cell carcinoma of the lung (Eaton-Lambert syndrome) and some patients in whom no malignancy is found. The chief symptom is weakness of proximal muscles in the limbs, especially of the pelvic girdles and thighs, which may improve at the start of exercise but soon returns after which the patient fatigues. There may be a mild bilateral ptosis but ocular and bulbar muscles are rarely involved. Deep tendon reflexes are usually depressed or absent.

In contrast to myasthenia gravis the response to edrophonium and other anticholinesterase drugs is poor. Again in contrast to myasthenia gravis the characteristic response to repetitive stimulation is an increase in size of an initially reduced compound muscle action potential. The mepps are of normal amplitude but reduced in frequency, and the number of quanta of acetylcholine released by a nerve impulse is greatly reduced. There is an IgG antibody to an antigen in the prejunctional nerve terminals, probably in the calcium channels.

Anticholinesterase drugs are relatively ineffective in treatment. Drugs that increase acetylcholine release (e.g. calcium, guanidine and 3,4-diaminopyridine) may be effective.

References

Engel. A. G. (1984) Myasthenia gravis and myasthenic syndromes. *Ann. Neurol.* **16**, 519–34.

Newsom Davis J. (1986) Diseases of the neuromuscular junction. In: *Diseases of the Nervous System*, Vol. 1, pp. 269–82. Eds A. K. Asbury, G. M. McKhann and W. I. McDonald, W. B. Saunders, Philadelphia.

Walton J. N. (1981) *Disorders of Voluntary Muscles*, 4th edn. Churchill-Livingstone, Edinburgh.

7 Autonomic Nervous System

The autonomic nervous system consists of two major divisions: the sympathetic (thoracolumbar division) and the parasympathetic (craniosacral outflow).

Sympathetic nervous system

Descending pathways from the hypothalamus and other regions of the brain synapse with cells of the preganglionic sympathetic efferents in the intermediolateral cell column of the spinal cord which extends from T1 to L2. The axons emerge in the spinal cord through the anterior roots which they leave via the white rami to join the sympathetic chain that consists of a series of ganglia and nerve fibres extending from the base of the skull to the coccyx. The preganglionic fibres, which enter the chain through the white rami, may synapse in the nearest ganglion, pass up or down the sympathetic chain before making their synapse, or pass through the chain to synapse at more peripheral ganglia such as the coeliac or other mesenteric ganglia. Postganglionic sympathetic fibres are unmyelinated; those that arise from the ganglia of the sympathetic chain join the main nerve trunks by way of the grey rami communicantes and are distributed to the sweat glands and blood vessels of skin and muscles (Fig. 7.1). The preganglionic sympathetic fibres are myelinated and cholinergic. The unmyelinated postganglionic fibres are noradrenergic, except those cholinergic fibres that innervate the sweat glands and some cholinergic vasodilator fibres to blood vessels in muscle. The release of peptides may play a role in the control of vasomotor tone and in the regulation of regional blood flow. Afferent fibres in the sympathetic nervous system convey mainly painful sensation.

Ocular sympathetic fibres leave the spinal cord in the first thoracic root and synapse in the superior cervical ganglion. Postganglionic fibres follow the course of the internal carotid artery to the siphon, where they join the ophthalmic division of the trigeminal nerve for distribution to the pupil. Interruption of these fibres causes ptosis and miosis on the affected side. Fibres responsible for sweating and vasomotor control in

Fig. 7.1 Schematic diagram of sympathetic nervous system showing preganglionic myelinated cholinergic fibres (—), postganglionic unmyelinated noradrenergic fibres (- - -) and postganglionic unmyelinated cholinergic fibres (●—●). (From Lance and McLeod, 1981, with permission of Butterworths, London.)

the face accompany the second and third thoracic nerve roots. After synapsing in the superior cervical ganglion they are distributed along the carotid artery in the periarterial plexus before passing to the skin along peripheral branches of the trigeminal nerve. Sympathetic deficit in the face is characterized by impairment of sweating and vasomotor control as well as ptosis and miosis (Horner's syndrome) (see p.136).

Parasympathetic nervous system

The hypothalamus and other centres in the brain maintain control over the divisions of the parasympathetic nervous system. Parasympathetic fibres leave the brainstem in the third, seventh, ninth, and tenth cranial nerves, and the spinal cord in the second, third and fourth sacral nerves. Parasympathetic fibres in the third cranial nerve supply the pupillary and ciliary muscles; those in the seventh cranial nerve supply the lacrimal, submandibular and sublingual glands through branches of the greater superficial petrosal and chorda tympani nerves (Fig. 7.2). The parotid gland is supplied by parasympathetic fibres in the ninth cranial nerve; the vagus nerve innervates the thoracic and abdominal viscera; the sacral outflow supplies the bladder and genital system and the large bowel. The ganglia lie close to the innervated structures so that the

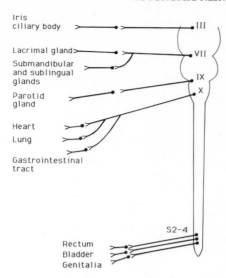

Fig. 7.2 Schematic diagram of parasympathetic nervous system. (From Lance and McLeod, 1981, with permission of Butterworths, London.)

postganglionic fibres are short. Both pre and postganglionic fibres in the parasympathetic nervous system are cholinergic.

Physiological functions of the autonomic nervous system

The most important clinical functions of the autonomic nervous system are control of blood pressure and heart rate, sweating, bladder and bowel (Chapter 8) and pupillary reflexes (Chapter 9).

Blood pressure and heart rate are controlled by baroreflex pathways (Fig. 7.3). Sensitive receptors in the carotid sinus, aortic arch and other thoracic regions respond to alterations in blood pressure. Afferent fibres from the baroreceptors in the carotid sinus run in the glossopharyngeal nerve and those from the aortic arch and thoracic low pressure receptors run in the vagus nerve. They synapse in the nucleus of the tractus solitarius and elsewhere in the brainstem and efferent fibres run in the vagus nerve to the heart and in the sympathetic nerves to the heart, mesenteric vascular bed and blood vessels in the skin and muscles. A rise in systemic blood pressure results in slowing of the heart and peripheral vasodilatation; a fall in blood pressure causes increased heart rate and peripheral vasoconstriction. The splanchnic vascular bed plays an im-

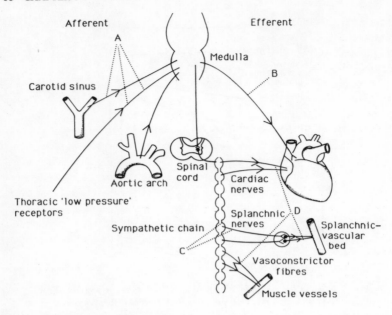

Fig. 7.3 Schematic representation of baroreflex pathways that control blood pressure and heart rate. (A) Afferent fibres from baroreceptors; (B) cardiac vagal efferent fibres; (C) preganglionic sympathetic efferent fibres; (D) postganglionic sympathetic efferent fibres. (From McLeod and Tuck, 1987.)

portant part in human blood pressure regulation. On standing, about 700 ml of blood leaves the chest and pools in the abdomen and legs, but as a result of reflex vasoconstriction in the splanchnic vascular bed and skeletal muscle vessels, blood is redistributed thus maintaining normal blood pressure.

Control of sweating The sweat glands are innervated mainly by cholinergic postganglionic sympathetic nerve fibres and are under hypothalamic control.

Disorders of autonomic function

The most important clinical manifestations of autonomic dysfunction are postural or orthostatic hypotension, impotence, disorders of bladder function, abnormalities of sweating, and vasomotor disturbances.

Patients with postural hypotension feel light-headed, dizzy or faint or lose consciousness on standing upright. Postural hypotension may result from dehydration or loss of blood, effects of drugs and other causes (see Chapter 17), or from diseases of the autonomic nervous system. These may affect central autonomic control or the peripheral autonomic pathways (Table 7.1).

Progressive autonomic failure, or *idiopathic orthostatic hypotension,* is a degenerative disorder which causes progressive loss of cells of origin of the preganglionic sympathetic fibres in the intermediolateral columns of the spinal cord. It may sometimes be associated with Parkinsonian features. It is more common in males and the usual age of onset is between 40 and 60 years. The earliest symptoms are those of postural hypotension with dizziness and weakness on standing or walking. Impotence, bladder disturbances and loss of sweating ability are common features. The condition is slowly progressive. Progressive autonomic failure may also be associated with a *multisystem atrophy* comprising pyramidal, extrapyramidal and cerebellar features in addition to profound postural hypotension *(Shy-Drager syndrome).*

Peripheral autonomic fibres may be damaged in peripheral neuropathies particularly those that affect small myelinated and unmyelinated fibres (e.g. diabetes, primary amyloidosis), or those which cause acute demyelination of the preganglionic sympathetic fibres and the vagal afferent and efferent fibres (e.g. Guillain-Barré syndrome). Postural hypotension, impairment of heart rate control, loss of sweating and impotence are the usual clinical manifestations. Autonomic neuropathy is particularly common in diabetes.

Tests of autonomic function

There is a large number of tests of autonomic function. They include the following.

Alteration of blood pressure with posture   There is normally little alteration of blood pressure on changing from the supine to the standing position. A fall of greater than 30/15 mmHg is regarded as significant.

Change of heart rate with posture   The heart rate normally increases by about 11–29 beats/min on changing from the supine to the standing position, reaching a maximum after 15 beats. There is then a reflex bradycardia which reaches its maximum at about the thirtieth beat. The ratio of the heart period, or R–R interval, on an ECG corresponding to the thirtieth and fifteenth heart beats, is known as the 30 : 15 ratio; the normal ratio varies with age. In autonomic neuropathies affecting the afferent or efferent fibres of the reflex arc the 30 : 15 ratio and the rise in heart rate with change in position are reduced.

Table 7.1   Classification of autonomic disorders

I. Diseases affecting central nervous system
    A. Progressive autonomic failure (PAF) (idiopathic orthostatic hypotension)
        1. Pure PAF
        2. PAF with parkinsonian features
        3. PAF with multiple-system atrophy (Shy-Drager syndrome)
    B. Parkinson's disease
    C. Spinal cord lesions
    D. Wernicke's encephalopathy
    E. Miscellaneous diseases
        1. Cerebrovascular disease
        2. Brainstem tumours
        3. Multiple sclerosis
        4. Adie's syndrome
        5. Tabes dorsalis

II. Diseases affecting the peripheral autonomic nervous system
    A. Disorders with no associated peripheral neuropathy
        1. Acute and subacute autonomic neuropathy
            a. Pandysautonomia
            b. Cholinergic dysautonomia
        2. Botulism
    B. Disorders associated with peripheral neuropathy
        1. Autonomic dysfunction, clinically important
            a. Diabetes
            b. Amyloidosis
            c. Acute inflammatory neuropathy (Guillain-Barré syndrome)
            d. Acute intermittent porphyria
            e. Familial dysautonomia (Riley-Day syndrome; HMSN III)
            f. Chronic sensory and autonomic neuropathy
        2. Autonomic dysfunction, usually clinically unimportant
            a. Alcohol-induced neuropathy
            b. Toxic neuropathies (vincristine sulfate, acrylamide, heavy metals, perhexiline maleate, organic solvents)
            c. HMSN I, II, and V
            d. Malignancy
            e. Vitamin B_{12} deficiency
            f. Rheumatoid arthritis
            g. Chronic renal failure
            h. Systemic lupus erythematosus
            i. Mixed connective tissue disease
            j. Fabry's disease
            k. Chronic inflammatory neuropathy

Change of heart rate with respiration During quiet respiration the heart rate increases during inspiration and decreases during expiration (sinus arrhythmia). In autonomic disturbances affecting the vagus nerve the heart rate variation with respiration is impaired.

Isometric contraction Sustained isometric contraction (e.g. a firm handgrip on a spring) for up to 5 min results in an increase in heart rate and systolic and diastolic blood pressure. The blood pressure rises because of increased cardiac output and peripheral vasoconstriction. The normal rise in diastolic blood pressure is 15 mmHg or more, and the response is impaired in diseases affecting sympathetic efferent fibres.

Response to emotional and other stimuli Mental arithmetic, a loud noise, or cold or painful stimuli applied to the body, will all increase the arterial blood pressure due to peripheral vasoconstriction. The reflex response is impaired in lesions of the sympathetic efferent pathways but may also be absent in some normal people.

Valsalva manoeuvre The heart rate and blood pressure normally change during and after the performance of a Valsalva manoeuvre (forced expiration against a closed glottis or mouthpiece; Fig. 7.4). The subject is asked to maintain a column of mercury at 40 mm pressure for 10–15 s while in a semi-recumbent posture. The ECG is monitored continuously and the blood pressure may be recorded through an intra-arterial catheter. The Valsalva ratio is the ratio of the longest pulse interval to the shortest pulse interval recorded on the ECG during the manoeuvre. In normal young adults it exceeds 1.45 and is impaired by diseases that affect the parasympathetic and sympathetic pathways.

Sweating Sweating is usually impaired in autonomic disorders affecting the sympathetic efferent pathways. The usual test is to cover the skin with a powder such as quinizarin or alazarine red that change colour when sweating occurs. The patient is warmed by a heat cradle, raising the body temperature by 1°C. Local sweating may also be tested by injection or iontophoresis of acetylcholine which stimulates an axon reflex, or pilocarpine which stimulates the sweat glands directly.

Pupillary responses Instillation of 2.5% methacholine (Mecholyl) into the conjunctival sac does not affect the size of the normal pupil but causes pupillary constriction if there are lesions of the parasympathetic innervation, because of the denervation supersensitivity of the constrictor muscle of the pupil.

I   II   III   IV

100 mmHg

10 s

Fig. 7.4 (A) Valsalva response from control subject; (B) Valsalva response from patient with primary amyloidosis. Arrows indicate onset and cessation of the Valsalva manoeuvre. Note in (B) the pronounced fall in mean arterial pressure in phase II, absence of bradycardia and absence of overshoot of blood pressure in phase IV. (From McLeod and Tuck, 1987.)

Instillation of 0.1% adrenaline has no effect on the normal pupil but causes dilatation of the pupil if postganglionic sympathetic innervation has been interrupted, because of denervation supersensitivity.

Cocaine blocks the re-uptake of noradrenaline so that 4% cocaine eye-drops cause dilatation of the normal pupil. If there has been interruption of the peripheral sympathetic innervation, pupillary dilatation does not occur.

Tyramine releases noradrenaline from peripheral nerve terminals so that 2% tyramine eye-drops produce pupillary dilatation. The reaction is impaired if there is noradrenaline depletion secondary to a sympathetic lesion.

Other tests of autonomic function   There are a number of other tests of vasomotor control and baroreflex sensitivity, as well as tests of bladder control, which are more difficult to perform. The tests referred to above can for the most part be performed relatively simply at the bedside.

References

Appenzeller O. (1982) *The Autonomic Nervous System*, 3rd edn, pp. 524. Elsevier, Amsterdam.

Bannister R. (ed.) (1988) *Autonomic Failure*, 2nd edn. Oxford University Press, Oxford.

Johnson R. H. and Spalding J. M. R. (1974) *Disorders of the Autonomic Nervous System*. Blackwell Scientific Publication, Oxford.

McLeod J. G. and Tuck R. R. (1987) Disorders of the autonomic nervous system. *Ann. Neurol.* **21**, 419–30; 519–29.

8 Spinal Cord

Anatomy

The spinal cord in adults extends from the foramen magnum to the upper border of the second lumbar vertebra (L2) (Fig. 8.1). The conus medullaris is the conical or inferior end of the cord from the apex of which a delicate filament, the filum terminale, extends and attaches to the first segment of the coccyx. The dura mater extends down to the level of the second sacral vertebra (S2) where it ends as a blind sac. The arachnoid also extends to the level of S2. The spinal fluid is contained in the subarachnoid space, and since the spinal cord ends at the L2 level lumbar puncture can be safely performed at the L3 and L4 level (usually L3-4 interspace) to obtain a sample of cerebrospinal fluid.

Fig. 8.1 Spinal cord and roots. (After Shadé, 1966, *The Peripheral Nervous System*. Elsevier Publishing Company, Amsterdam.)

Thirty-one pairs of roots (cervical, thoracic, lumbar, sacral and coccygeal) arise from the spinal cord, each with its ventral (anterior) and dorsal (posterior) root. The dorsal root ganglion is a swelling on the dorsal root which contains the cell bodies of afferent nerve fibres. The roots pass at an increasingly oblique angle to progressively lower levels of the spinal cord. In the lumbosacral region they descend almost vertically as the *cauda equina*.

Ventral roots contain efferent fibres originating in anterior and lateral grey columns, and also some afferent fibres. Dorsal roots contain afferent fibres originating in dorsal root ganglia.

When interpreting clinical signs of spinal cord disease it is important to remember the following anatomical points:

(1) The corticospinal tracts cross from the contralateral motor cortex to the opposite side in the lower medulla so that spinal cord damage will cause a motor deficit on the same side (Figs 3.1, 3.2).

(2) When sensory fibres enter the spinal cord from the dorsal roots:

(a) large diameter fibres conveying proprioceptive information pass up the dorsal columns on the same side (Fig. 4.3);

(b) small myelinated and unmyelinated fibres conveying pain and temperature sensation synapse in the dorsal horn of the grey matter within a few segments of their entry, and the second order neurones cross to the other side and ascend in the lateral spinothalamic tract (Fig. 4.2);

(c) most fibres conveying the sensation of light touch pass uncrossed up the dorsal columns but some cross and ascend in the ventral spinothalamic tracts (Fig. 4.3). Because of this bilateral representation, unilateral spinal cord lesions do not usually completely destroy the sense of touch.

Blood supply of the spinal cord

The largest arterial supply is the *anterior spinal artery* which is formed by the union of paired branches of the vertebrals and passes along the anterior surface of the cord, narrowing near the upper fourth thoracic segment at which level a watershed area exists. Below T4 there is a segmental supply from the intercostal arteries from the aorta; the longest of these branches — the great ventral radicular artery (artery of Adamkiewicz) — enters between T8 and L4 (Fig. 8.2).

At the lumbosacral level radicular arteries are derived from larger regional vessels; the largest such vessel enters the intervertebral foramen at L2 to form the lowermost portion of the anterior spinal artery — the terminal artery — which runs along the filum terminale. Posterior spinal arteries are paired and considerably smaller than the anterior spinal

Fig. 8.2 Blood supply of the spinal cord. Shaded area is that supplied by anterior spinal artery. (After Henson and Parsons, 1967.)

vessels. They receive branches from the posterolateral plexus at various levels.

The anterior spinal artery supplies the anterior and lateral columns on either side. The posterior spinal arteries supply the posterior white columns and part of the posterior grey columns (Fig. 8.2).

Occlusion of the anterior spinal artery affects the corticospinal and spinothalamic tracts but usually spares the dorsal columns (Fig. 8.2).

General clinical features of spinal cord injury

Damage to the spinal cord may produce motor, sensory and autonomic signs.

Motor signs

Motor signs follow damage to corticospinal tracts or anterior horn cells, resulting in paralysis of the upper motor neurone type below the lesion (corticospinal tract) and of the lower motor neurone type at the level of the lesion (anterior horn cell). Damage below the conus medullaris, i.e. to the cauda equina, will cause only lower motor neurone signs.

Sensory signs

Sensory signs result from damage to the sensory pathways within the spinal cord, or to the dorsal roots or ganglia. An anteriorly placed lesion, such as thrombosis of the anterior spinal artery, will affect the spino-thalamic sensory pathways (pain and temperature) but not dorsal columns (joint position, two-point discrimination, vibration sense). This impairment of pain and temperature with sparing of other modalities is called dissociated sensory loss. Because of the lamination of fibres entering the spinal cord, certain cutaneous areas may escape from sensory loss, since a compressive lesion affects mainly the outer layers. Thus it is common for sacral areas to be spared ('sacral sparing').

Compression of dorsal roots at the level of the lesion may result in a band of hyperaesthesia and hyperalgesia, but anaesthesia or analgesia may later follow.

The spine may be tender to pressure or percussion in disease of the vertebrae (e.g. inflammation), or after damage to the spinal cord or roots which innervate the same level as the vertebra.

Autonomic signs

Autonomic disturbances may occur below the level of a spinal cord lesion; the skin becomes warm and dry, and there is loss of pilomotor reaction and of vasomotor tone. Bladder, bowel and sexual function may be impaired.

Clinical approach to patients with spinal cord lesions

The questions that need to be asked in a patient presenting with a spinal cord lesion are:

(a) What is the level of the lesion? Is the lesion localized, multiple or diffuse?

(b) What is the nature of the lesion?

(c) Is it surgically remediable?

These questions can usually be answered after a careful history has been taken, a systematic physical examination has been performed, and appropriate investigations have been carried out.

History

The patient may complain of girdle pains in thoracic lesions; of tingling in the spine, fingers and toes on flexing the neck (Lhermitte's sign) in cervical lesions; of pain in the shoulders and weakness in hands in cervical cord lesions; or of weakness in legs or difficulty in micturition at any level of cord lesions. An analysis of symptoms may help indicate the approximate level of the lesion. Root pain occurs especially with extramedullary lesions such as prolapsed intervertebral discs or neurofibromas.

Examination

A full examination with attention to distribution of muscle wasting or weakness, reflex changes, sensory levels and autonomic changes, usually will enable the level of the lesion to be localized. It is most important to determine accurately the level of the lesion. The spine should be palpated and percussed to elicit local or referred pain. Listen for a bruit if an angioma is suspected. Do not forget to look for signs on general examination which may reveal the nature of the underlying disorder, e.g. a hard prostate or lump in the breast (carcinoma with metastases), lymphadenopathy (reticuloses, carcinoma), smooth red tongue (pernicious anaemia), *café au lait* patches on the skin (neurofibromatosis), or cutaneous angioma.

Special investigations

(a) Plain X-ray of the appropriate area of the spine. Reduction of intervertebral disc spaces, narrowing of intervertebral foramina, and osteophyte formation, indicate degeneration of the spine. Destruction or collapse of vertebrae may be seen with myeloma, metastases and infections; erosion of pedicles is a sign of an extramedullary tumour.

(b) Chest X-ray, to exclude malignancy, lymphoma, tuberculosis.

(c) CT scan of the spine.

(d) Myelogram, specifying in your request the level at which the lesion is suspected. A radio-opaque contrast medium is injected into the lumbar or cisternal subarachnoid space and tumours, disc protrusions and other causes of spinal cord or root compression can be delineated radiologically. Myelography is most informative if followed by CT scan. Cerebrospinal fluid should be taken at the time of myelography and examined with particular regard to protein content, IgG/albumin ratio, and presence of oligoclonal bands on electrophoresis if multiple sclerosis is suspected. Serological tests should be done if syphilis is suspected.

(e) Magnetic resonance imaging (MRI) gives clear sagittal views of vertebrae, discs, and cord, that may obviate the need for myelography and may demonstrate intrinsic lesions such as syringomyelia.

(f) Other routine investigations such as full blood count and ESR.

Spinal cord compression

Compression of the spinal cord may be caused by:
(a) Disease of the vertebral column, e.g. secondary carcinoma, tuberculosis, osteomyelitis, prolapsed disc.
(b) Lesions inside the spinal canal.
Extramedullary causes — (i) Extradural. These often cause local pain and tenderness, are usually rapidly progressive and cause bilateral signs, e.g. secondary tumour, extradural abscess, haematoma, lymphoma, hydatid cyst. (ii) Intradural. These are often benign and more slowly progressive. They may be predominantly unilateral, e.g. meningioma, neurofibroma, lipoma.
Intramedullary causes — these usually do not cause radicular pain, e.g. ependymoma, glioma, syringomyelia.

Symptoms and signs of spinal cord compression

The specific clinical features depend on the nature and extent of the spinal cord lesion. In general, clinical features of spinal cord compression at a given level consist of: (i) lower motor neurone lesion at the segmental level of compression; (ii) upper motor neurone lesion below the level of compression; (iii) dorsal root irritation at the segmental level of compression; (iv) sensory loss below the level of compression with a distinct upper level; (v) autonomic changes (e.g. excessive sweating) below the level of the lesion.

Complete transection   This usually results from trauma. Initially there is a state of spinal shock with a flaccid paralysis and loss of all sensation and reflexes below the lesion [paraplegia, if lower limbs only affected; quadriplegia (tetraplegia) if all four limbs are involved]. The loss of reflexes and hypotonia are due to depression of alpha and gamma motoneurone activity. Reflex bladder and bowel function are suppressed and acute painless retention occurs. Below the level of the lesion autonomic changes may be seen; the skin is warm and dry and there is loss of pilomotor reaction and vasomotor tone.

The state of spinal shock passes after approximately 3 weeks and reflexes become brisk. Muscle tone is restored in the limbs especially in flexor muscle groups. A flexor withdrawal reflex may result from noxious stimuli applied to the skin below the level of the lesion. The reflexes are heightened because of recovery of gamma motoneurone function and alpha motoneurone hyperexcitability.

Incomplete or partial lesions   Partial spinal cord lesions may be due to trauma, tumours and other conditions. An early symptom of a spinal cord lesion is precipitancy or urgency of micturition which may later, in the case of expanding tumours and multiple sclerosis, progress to incontinence or retention of urine. Weakness of the lower limbs (spastic paraparesis) is usually present. Muscle tone and deep tendon reflexes in the lower limbs are increased, plantar responses become extensor, and a sensory level may be detected on the trunk.

Hemisection of spinal cord   Hemisection is rarely precise; an incomplete syndrome is more frequently seen. A pure hemisection causes Brown-Séquard syndrome (Fig. 8.3) which is characterized by:
(a) Ipsilateral paralysis of the upper motor neurone type below the lesion, with lower motor neurone signs at the level of the lesion.
(b) Ipsilateral loss of tactile sensation, joint position sense, two-point discrimination and vibration sense below the level of the lesion because of injury to the dorsal columns.
(c) Contralateral loss of pain and temperature sensation below the level of the lesion as a result of damage to the spinothalamic tracts. Spino-

Fig. 8.3 Clinical features resulting from hemisection of the spinal cord (Brown-Séquard syndrome). (After Walshe, 1963, *Diseases of the Nervous System*, 10th edn, E & S Livingstone, Edinburgh and London.)

Fig. 8.4 Segmental overlap of pain fibres entering the spinal cord. A transverse lesion may result in sensory change one or two segments below the level of the lesion.

thalamic fibres cross to the opposite side within a few segments of entering the cord and thus it is usual to find that the level of contralateral spinothalamic sensory change is a few segments below the level of the causative lesion (Fig. 8.4). There may be some ipsilateral impairment of pain and temperature sense at the level of the lesion because of interruption of the fibres at the dorsal root entry zone.

This pattern of abnormal signs (upper and lower motor neurone signs and sensory abnormalities with a distinct upper level) is seen in various forms wherever the spinal cord is compressed.

Cervical spondylosis

Cervical spondylosis is characterized by osteophyte formation, disc degeneration and disc protrusion (Fig. 8.5). These abnormalities cause

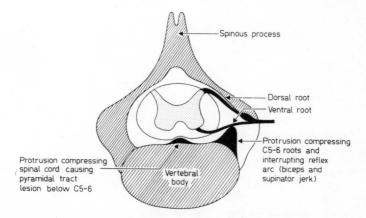

Fig. 8.5 Mechanism of reflex changes in cervical spondylosis at C5–6 level.

compression of nerve roots, and of the spinal cord and its blood supply. Although it may occur at other levels (particularly C4–5 and C6–7) the most common site of pathology is at C5–6, the clinical features of which are: (a) pain in neck and shoulders; (b) wasting of deltoid, biceps or brachioradialis muscles (C5–6); (c) exaggerated reflexes in lower limbs (corticospinal tract involvement); (d) depression of C5–6 reflexes (i.e. biceps, brachioradialis), and exaggeration of triceps jerk (C7) and finger flexion (C8) reflexes. This combination of reflex changes is sometimes referred to as the 'inverted supinator reflex' (Fig. 8.6); sensory changes may not be prominent, but if present occur over the C5–6 dermatomes.

Fig. 8.6 The 'inverted supinator jerk'. Percussion of the radius sets up a vibration wave as in Fig. 3.5. When reflex arcs employing the fifth and sixth cervical segments are interrupted by disease, the biceps and brachioradialis responses to the vibration wave are absent (O). If the spinal cord is also compressed at the C5–6 level, reflexes below that level such as the triceps jerk (C7 segment) and finger jerk (C8 segment) may be enhanced so that the elbow extends while the fingers flex. (From Lance and McLeod, 1981, with permission of Butterworths, London.)

Cauda equina and lumbosacral root lesions

One of the most common causes of compression of the *cauda equina* is a protruding lumbar disc. Other causes include neoplasms, arachnoiditis and cysts. Pain is usually a prominent feature.

The most common cause of an isolated lumbosacral root lesion is an intervertebral disc protrusion, usually at L4–5 or L5–S1 levels. The main clinical features are:

Pain   This is felt in the back and radiates down the back of the leg to: the heel and lateral border of the foot if the S1 root is compressed; the lateral aspect of the leg, lateral malleolus and dorsum of the foot if L5 is the main root involved; and the thigh, knee and medial malleolus and sometimes the groin if the L4 root is compressed. The pain is made worse by coughing, sneezing, straining, bending and stooping.

Weakness and wasting   L4 involvement results in wasting and weakness of quadriceps, tibialis anterior (dorsiflexion of foot) and tibialis posterior (inversion of foot) and depression of the knee jerk. L5 lesions cause weakness of the extensor hallucis longus (dorsiflexion of the big toe); and S1 lesions cause wasting of calf and extensor digitorum brevis muscles, intrinsic foot muscles, weakness of eversion (peroneus longus) and plantar flexion (gastrocnemius), and absent ankle jerk.

Larger disc protrusions or neoplasms can cause more extensive muscle wasting, weakness and sensory loss. There may be loss of sensation in the perineal region (saddle anaesthesia) when lower sacral roots are involved.

Disturbance of bowel and bladder function usually occurs later but may occasionally be the presenting symptom and is caused by direct involvement of S2–4 roots. Signs of an upper motor neurone lesion indicate that the spinal cord is involved above the conus medullaris.

Conus medullaris lesions

Tumours which invade the lowermost part of the cord (conus medullaris) may involve the roots as well as producing cord signs. Bowel and bladder function are affected early. The signs are similar to those of cauda equina lesions, although brisk ankle jerks and extensor plantar responses may also be present if the lesion extends above the conus.

Other conditions which may give rise to symptomatology related to the spinal cord

Acute lesions

Anterior spinal artery thrombosis   The blood supply to the cord may become impaired as a result of atherosclerosis, hypotension, emboli or surgical interference, causing infarction most commonly about the T4 level (see p. 95–6).

Occlusion of the anterior spinal artery affects the anterior horns and the corticospinal and spinothalamic tracts, but usually spares the dorsal columns (Fig. 8.2).

Transverse myelitis   The onset is usually acute or subacute, often with pain. There may be a flaccid paralysis, a well defined sensory level and sphincter disturbance. The condition may be of viral or demyelinating aetiology.

Chronic lesions

The pattern of spinal cord degeneration in some chronic conditions is shown diagrammatically in Fig. 8.7.

Syringomyelia   This disorder is characterized by cystic dilatation in the spinal cord surrounded by gliosis, usually in the lower cervical and upper thoracic region. The cystic dilatation forms a cavity (syrinx) in the cord.

The anterior horn cells degenerate as a result of compression by the cyst causing muscle wasting and weakness usually first seen in the small hand muscles. If the syrinx extends into the medulla, the nucleus ambiguus and hypoglossal nuclei are affected, resulting in wasting and weakness of the tongue, soft palate, pharynx, and vocal cords. When the corticospinal tracts become involved, the lower limbs become spastic. Reflexes are lost over the affected segments of the cord.

The crossing pain and temperature fibres destined for the lateral spinothalamic tracts become interrupted causing loss of pain and temperature sense in one or two segments in the upper limbs or in a cape-like distribution across the back and shoulders. Touch and position sense are retained initially (*dissociated sensory loss*) but later the dorsal columns may also be involved. Patients often sustain burns without feeling them and scars may be seen on their hands. Loss of pain and temperature sense over one side of the face may result from involvement of the spinal tract

Fig. 8.7 Pattern of degeneration (black areas) in the spinal cord in (1) syringomyelia; (2) amyotrophic lateral sclerosis; (3) tabes dorsalis; (4) subacute combined degeneration; (5) Friedreich's ataxia; (6) multiple sclerosis. ST, spinothalamic tract; CST, corticospinal tract; AHC, anterior horn cells; VR, ventral root; DC, dorsal columns; DRG, dorsal root ganglion; SCT, spinocerebellar tracts.

of the Vth nerve. Trophic changes in the extremities give rise to a soft fleshy appearance of the fingers and Charcot joints.

Motor neurone disease (amyotrophic lateral sclerosis) (see pp. 278–9)   This disease occurs most commonly between the ages of 40 and 60 years, and is characterized pathologically by degenerative changes most marked in the anterior horn cells of the spinal cord, the motor nuclei of the medulla, and the corticospinal tracts. There is therefore degeneration of both the upper and lower motor neurones, but no involvement of sensory pathways.

Tabes dorsalis (see Chapter 19)   Tabes dorsalis is a form of tertiary syphilis. The patients may experience lightning (stabbing), pains. The pathological changes are those of degeneration of dorsal roots and of fibres in the dorsal columns. Hypotonia and loss of reflexes result from damage to the dorsal roots and interruption of the stretch reflex arc.

There is often patchy loss of painful sensation over the sternum, tibial prominences and the bridge of the nose; and impairment of position and vibration sense. Deep pain sensation may be lost, and in about 10% of patients this results in painless destruction of weight-bearing joints (Charcot joints). This arthropathy is seen in other neurological conditions in which central or peripheral pain pathways are damaged (e.g. syringomyelia, diabetes, hereditary sensory neuropathy). There is no primary motor involvement. Plantar reflexes are usually flexor. The gait is high stepping. Retention of urine with a painless overdistended bladder is common. Argyll Robertson pupils (see pp. 134–5) occur in about 90% of cases.

Subacute combined degeneration   Subacute combined degeneration results from Vitamin B_{12} deficiency, and is usually seen in pernicious anaemia and malabsorption states. The peripheral nerves and brain may be affected, and dorsal columns, corticospinal tracts and spinocerebellar tracts degenerate.

The condition usually presents with paraesthesiae, consisting of tingling sensations in fingers and toes, and the lower limbs become weak as a result of an upper motor neurone lesion combined with peripheral neuropathy. Position and vibration sense are usually markedly impaired. There may be a glove-and-stocking type of anaesthesia caused by the associated peripheral neuropathy. Romberg's sign may be positive. Reflexes may be depressed or increased depending on the degree of peripheral nerve involvement. Plantar reflexes are often extensor. Incoordination may be marked. Lower motor neurone signs are absent, unless peripheral neuropathy is severe. Mental confusion, dementia, and optic atrophy may occur.

There may be signs of glossitis, or anaemia, but it is important to remember that the neurological features may be present with a normal peripheral blood count. The serum Vitamin B_{12} level should always be measured if this diagnosis is suspected because the condition is potentially reversible.

Friedreich's ataxia (see p. 281)   Friedreich's ataxia is a disease with an autosomal recessive inheritance. It usually presents in the second or third decade of life with ataxia, dysarthria, and incoordination. Pathologically, there is degeneration of the dorsal columns, corticospinal and spinocerebellar tracts, and dorsal root ganglia and peripheral nerves.

Clinically, slurred speech, nystagmus, ataxia, and incoordination are usually present. Reflexes are depressed or absent because of dorsal root involvement. Position and vibration sense are impaired. Plantar responses are extensor. In addition, there are usually associated skeletal deformities such as kyphoscoliosis and pes cavus. Cardiomyopathy is common.

Multiple sclerosis (see Chapter 20)   Multiple sclerosis, which usually starts in young adult life, is characterized by the occurrence of plaques of demyelination at different levels in the white matter of the central nervous system.

The lesions are disseminated in both time and space, and involvement of the optic nerves, spinal cord and brainstem may occur at different times.

When a plaque of demyelination affects the spinal cord, it usually presents as a transverse lesion. There may be spasticity below the level of the lesion and sensory loss with a well-defined upper border. Bladder involvement is the rule.

To be sure of the diagnosis, one should have clinical evidence from history and examination of lesions elsewhere in the nervous system. Otherwise compressive spinal cord lesions must be excluded by appropriate investigations.

Innervation and nervous control of the urinary bladder

The structure of the bladder

The bladder is composed of smooth muscle fibres in three layers — outer and inner longitudinal layers, and a middle circular layer. The fibres form a continuum, and act as a functional whole called the detrusor muscle of the bladder. The smooth muscle fibres around the internal orifice of the urethra form the internal sphincter. It is not a separate anatomical structure, but is simply part of the detrusor and has no separate innervation. On the other hand the external sphincter muscle is a separate structure and consists of striated muscle fibres.

Innervation of the bladder

The smooth muscle of the bladder is innervated by sympathetic and parasympathetic fibres, while the external sphincter receives only somatic innervation (Fig. 8.8).

Efferent

Parasympathetic innervation   Preganglionic fibres arise from grey matter of sacral cord segments S2–4, and travel in pelvic nerves to form a diffuse subserosal network in the bladder wall. Postganglionic fibres innervate the smooth muscle fibres. Parasympathetic efferent impulses cause the detrusor muscles to contract and the bladder neck to shorten thus allowing the passage of urine.

Fig. 8.8 Innervation of the urinary bladder. ——— Efferent fibres; ---- afferent fibres. (From Lance and McLeod, 1981, with permission of Butterworths, London.)

Sympathetic innervation　Preganglionic fibres arise from the intermediolateral columns in the T11–L2 segments of the spinal cord and travel via the ventral roots and white rami to the hypogastric plexus. Postganglionic fibres join the subserosal plexus on the bladder wall and seem to go mainly to the trigone and the neck of the bladder rather than to the whole detrusor muscle. Sympathetic efferents may inhibit the detrusor but appear to play little part in the act of micturition.

Somatic innervation　The pudendal nerve (S2–4) supplies the external sphincter. Its action is coordinated with the detrusor, and it is relaxed during micturition. It can also be voluntarily contracted to terminate the act of micturition.

Afferent

Free and encapsulated nerve endings have been demonstrated in the bladder wall.

Parasympathetic fibres   These fibres transmit sensations of bladder full-ness, pain, overdistension and overcontraction. They also mediate the reflex for bladder contraction through S2–4 segments.

Sympathetic fibres   These fibres convey painful sensation from the tri-gone area, and a vague sensation of bladder fullness. They play no part in the micturition reflex.

Somatic fibres   The somatic fibres in the pudendal nerve innervate the sphincter and urethra, and convey sensations of urine passing through the urethra and of bladder emptying.

Afferent connections within the central nervous system

Impulses giving rise to sensations of bladder fullness and the desire to micturate, the sensation of pain from the bladder, and pain and tem-perature from the urethra are mediated by lateral spinothalamic tracts. No thermal sensations can be elicited from the bladder.

Touch and pressure sense derived from the urethra and vague sen-sations of awareness of bladder fullness are mediated through the posterior columns (Fig. 8.9).

Supraspinal control of micturition

The higher centres inhibit the micturition reflex. Micturition is initiated by the removal of this tonic suprasegmental inhibition of the reflex arc. There are cortical centres in the region of the paracentral lobule, and also centres of influence in the hypothalamus and midbrain. Descending pathways course in the lateral columns of the spinal cord medial to the corticospinal tracts (Fig. 8.9).

Bladder tone

This is a property of the smooth muscle of the bladder wall and is un-related to the extrinsic innervation of the bladder. Thus spinal cord transection, and spinal anaesthesia do not directly influence bladder tone. The 'atonic bladder' described in spinal cord and sacral nerve injury is due to chronic overstretching of the bladder consequent upon the loss of the micturition reflex and is only an indirect result of de-nervation. The hypertonic or small contracted bladder is the result of inflammatory changes in the bladder wall — chronic cystitis — rather than of damage to the innervation of the bladder.

Fig. 8.9 Nervous control of the urinary bladder. Descending and ascending pathways in the spinal cord. (From Lance and McLeod, 1981, with permission of Butterworths, London.)

Micturition reflex

When the bladder is distended to a critical level, the stretch receptors in the wall initiate impulses in the afferent limb of the sacral reflex arc, causing contraction of the detrusor muscle through the parasympathetic efferents from the S2–4 segments. The micturition reflex is normally inhibited through the descending corticospinal pathway, and voluntary micturition is initiated by removal of suprasegmental inhibition.

The *cystometrogram* records the relationship of urine volume to intra-vesical pressure. The usual technique is to fill the bladder through a urethral catheter measuring both the pressure and volume of fluid. As the bladder is filled, the pressure increases gradually. Low-level rhythmical contractions, associated with a transient sense of urgency, usually develop at a volume of 150–200 ml and a sense of fullness at about 150–300 ml. Reflex micturition then starts with rhythmic waves of increasing amplitude, developing into a sustained contraction of the detrusor muscle.

Bladder dysfunction resulting from disease of the nervous system

Sacral dorsal root disease

Afferent fibres of the micturition reflex arc may be selectively damaged by peripheral neuropathy, tabes dorsalis, subacute combined degeneration, herpes zoster, or compression by a prolapsed lumbar disc or neoplasm. Initially the sense of bladder fullness may be impaired and the sense of urgency becomes less clear-cut. The bladder becomes overdistended, because of lack of sensation, and may contain huge volumes of urine (1500–2000 ml) with overflow incontinence. Abdominal compression may be necessary to empty the bladder. The cystometrogram reveals loss of tone from overdistension, a high threshold for filling sensation, and elevation of the threshold or abolition of the micturition reflex.

Sacral spinal cord and motor root disease

Peripheral neuropathy, cauda equina tumours, lumbar disc protrusion, or trauma may damage efferent sacral roots.

Poliomyelitis temporarily paralyses preganglionic autonomic neurones; and neoplasms, spinal injuries, or trauma may interrupt the micturition reflex arc in the spinal cord.

After acute lesions of the motor roots, bladder tone remains unaltered and the cystometrogram will demonstrate normal tone and rhythmic contractions. Bladder distension causes discomfort and painful fullness. Pain eventually remits and thereafter the features are similar to those of afferent sacral lesions.

If the bladder is allowed to remain overdistended for long periods it may fail to regain significant autonomous activity. The patient should therefore be catheterized and the bladder decompressed as soon as possible. After decompression, the bladder usually regains contractility and may become hyperactive. After 2–3 months, autonomous contractions become sufficiently strong to contract the detrusor and open the internal sphincter. Emptying is incomplete but may be aided by abdominal compression. Usually significant residual urine remains and the bladder becomes prone to infections.

Spinal cord injury

In slowly developing and partial lesions of the spinal cord (such as multiple sclerosis and compression by spinal tumours) there may be loss of descending inhibition, causing urgency and precipitancy of micturition with ejection of a small urine volume. As the lesion progresses, voluntary control of micturition may be totally impaired, causing retention of urine.

In acute spinal transection, descending nervous inhibition is over-whelming (spinal shock) and the micturition reflex is suppressed. Urinary retention and infection occur. After spinal shock has passed the micturition reflex may be facilitated.

Cerebral lesions

Loss of control of micturition may result from lesions of the motor cortex (paracentral lobules). Lesions of the frontal lobe may cause precipitancy and incontinence.

Innervation of the rectum

The nerve supply of the rectum is similar to that of the bladder, and micturition and defaecation are physiologically comparable.

Sexual functions

Erection of the penis may be reflex, mediated by the S2–3 segments, or of psychogenic origin. The reflex pathway may be tested by the bulbo-cavernosus response (squeezing the glans penis, or touching it firmly with a pin, which evokes a contraction of the bulbocavernosus muscle palpable at the base of the penis in the perineum). The reflex arc may be interrupted by any of the conditions discussed in relation to the micturition reflex and is particularly prone to damage in diabetes. Some cases of impotence are of psychogenic origin and the presence of the bulbocavernosus reflex together with a history of nocturnal or morning erections gives some reassurance that the reflex arc is intact.

Ejaculation into the urethra is a function of the sympathetic nervous system but ejaculation from the urethra requires activity of the bulbo-cavernosus muscle.

References

Henson R.A. and Parsons M. (1967) Ischaemic lesions of the spinal cord: an illustrated review. *Quart. J. Med.* **36**, 205–22.

Nyberg-Hansen R. (1966) Innervation and nervous control of the urinary bladder. *Acta Neurol. Scand.* Suppl. 20, **42**, 7–24.

Plum F. (1962) Bladder dysfunction. In *Modern Trends in Neurology* Vol. 3, pp. 151–72. Ed. D. Williams. Butterworths, London.

Van Arsdalen K.N. and Wein A.J. (1986) Micturition and bladder dysfunction. In *Diseases of the Nervous System*, pp. 618–25. Eds A.K. Asbury, G.M. McKhann and W.I. McDonald. W.B. Saunders, Philadelphia.

9 Cranial Nerves

I olfactory nerve

The olfactory portion of the nasal mucous membrane contains bipolar cells, the central processes of which form the olfactory filaments that pass through the cribriform plate to the olfactory bulb. The olfactory tract runs back and divides into medial and lateral olfactory striae; central connections are made in the prepyriform area, amygdala, and other structures.

The sense of smell is tested separately at each nostril with test odours, e.g. tobacco, coffee, peppermint, and cloves. Pungent and irritating test substances such as ammonia should be avoided.

Loss of sense of smell (anosmia) may result from: (i) local causes, e.g. colds, sinusitis, deviated nasal septum; (ii) head injury, with or without fracture of bone, causing damage to the olfactory filaments; (iii) meningiomas, gliomas and other tumours in the anterior cranial fossa which directly involve the olfactory bulb and central pathways; (iv) meningitis, acute or chronic, which damages the olfactory filaments.

II optic nerve

Light falls on the rods and cones of the retina, which lie on its outermost layer. Impulses are transmitted from these end-organs through a relay of bipolar cells to the ganglion cell fibres which enter the optic nerve.

The macula, on the temporal side of the optic disc, is the area of the retina specialized for central vision and the perception of detailed images; it has a high concentration of cones and contains no rods.

An object in the left temporal field of vision will cast an image on the right temporal and left nasal retinae. An object in the upper field of vision will cast an image on the inferior retinal quadrants.

Fibres from the temporal region of the retina course in the temporal half of the optic nerve, the upper temporal fibres lying in its upper temporal quadrant. The nasal half of the retina is represented in the

Fig. 9.1 Visual pathways.

nasal half of the optic nerve. The macular fibres occupy a central position (Fig. 9.1).

In the *optic chiasm* the nasal fibres from each retina cross while those from the temporal halves remain uncrossed. The crossed and uncrossed fibres unite to form the optic tracts (Fig. 9.1).

The anatomical relations of the optic chiasm are important (Figs 9.2, 9.3). Above it lies the cavity of the third ventricle and on its lateral aspects are the internal carotid arteries before they divide into anterior and middle cerebral vessels. Anterior to the chiasm lie the anterior cerebral vessels and the anterior communicating artery. Posteriorly lies the interpeduncular area, and below lies the pituitary gland in the sella turcica.

In the optic tracts, the fibres from the lower retinal quadrants are laterally placed and those from the upper retinal quadrants are medial.

The fibres from the optic tracts pass back to the *lateral geniculate body*, from where they relay to the *visual cortex* in the occipital lobes by way of

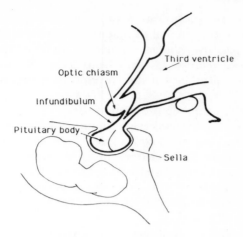

Fig. 9.2 Anatomical relations of the optic chiasm in the sagittal plane.

Fig. 9.3 Anatomical relations of the optic chiasm viewed from below.

the *optic radiation* (geniculo-calcarine tract) (Fig. 9.1). This tract is situated posteriorly in the internal capsule. The lowermost fibres of the optic radiation pass over the antero-superior aspect of the temporal horn of the lateral ventricle (Meyer's loop). These fibres are derived from the inferior quadrants of the corresponding hemiretinae (Fig. 9.4).

The remainder of the optic radiation passes through the parietal lobes close to the temporal and occipital horns of the lateral ventricle to terminate in the visual or striate cortex (area 17) which lies on either side of the calcarine fissure. The uppermost fibres of the optic radiation terminate in the upper lip (cuneus); the lowermost fibres terminate in the lower lip (lingual gyrus). The macular area is represented posteriorly, and the most peripheral parts of the retina are represented anteriorly in the visual cortex (Fig. 9.5).

The blood supply of the visual cortex is derived chiefly from the posterior cerebral artery, but the middle cerebral vessels may supply the tip of the occipital pole thus accounting for macular sparing in some cases of posterior cerebral artery occlusion.

The examination of the second cranial nerve includes testing of visual acuity, ophthalmoscopic examination and charting of the visual fields. It is described in detail in Chapter 2.

Anatomical classification of visual field defects

Some of the more common types of visual field defect are shown in Fig. 9.6.

Fig. 9.4 Optic radiation. (Modified from Ranson and Clark, 1959, *The Anatomy of the Nervous System*, 10th edn, W.B. Saunders, Philadelphia and London.)

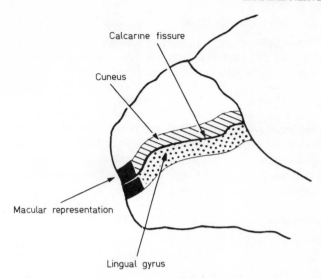

Fig. 9.5 Visual cortex. (Modified from Ranson and Clark, 1959, *The Anatomy of the Nervous System*, 10th edn, W.B. Saunders, Philadelphia and London.)

Fig 9.6 Field defects. (a) Right optic nerve lesion. (b) Right central scotoma e.g. retrobulbar neuritis. (c) Bitemporal hemianopia caused by a chiasmal lesion. (d) Right superior quandrantanopia resulting from a left temporal lobe lesion. (e) Right homonymous hemianopia from a deep left hemisphere or left occipital lobe lesion.

Retina

Detachment of the retina, retinitis pigmentosa, and glaucoma give rise to characteristic field defects. An island where vision is absent or defective is known as a 'scotoma'.

Optic nerve

In papilloedema (p. 119), the blind spot is increased in size and later the peripheral field becomes uniformly diminished.

In optic neuritis (p. 120), central or paracentral scotomata may develop. Complete lesions of the optic nerve result in total blindness of the affected eye.

Chiasmal lesions

The commonest lesions of the chiasm are those caused by pressure from tumours arising either in the pituitary fossa, or above the sella such as suprasellar cysts, craniopharyngiomas and meningiomas (Figs 9.2, 9.3). The chiasm may also be involved by gliomas, it may be compressed by the third ventricle in obstructive hydrocephalus (Fig. 9.2), or it may be compressed by an enlarging aneurysm on the nearby arteries (Fig. 9.3).

Pressure in the midline, initially involving crossing fibres, gives rise to a bitemporal hemianopia (Fig. 9.6). If pressure is from below, inferior nasal fibres will be involved first, giving a bitemporal superior quadrantanopia. If pressure is from above, an inferior quadrantanopia will result.

However, pressure effects from tumours are rarely symmetrical. Some tumours compress one optic nerve together with crossing fibres from the other eye, thus giving rise to a scotoma in one eye and a superior temporal quadrantanopia in the other. Asymmetry of the visual field defects is the rule in chiasmal lesions.

Optic tracts

The optic tracts may be compressed by pituitary tumours, temporal lobe tumours, aneurysms, and other expanding lesions. Homonymous hemianopia results, but it is usually incongruous (i.e. it is not bilaterally symmetrical) and incomplete.

Optic radiation

Lesions of the optic radiation result in homonymous field defects. Lesions in the temporal lobe may involve Meyer's loop, causing a superior homonymous quadrantanopia on the contralateral side (Fig. 9.6). Lesions in the parietal lobe may cause an inferior homonymous quadrantanopia or inattention to the opposite half-field. Complete homonymous hemianopia may result from a more extensive lesion.

When there is a lesion of the striate cortex of one occipital lobe, such as infarction following occlusion of one posterior cerebral artery, a contralateral symmetrical (congruous) homonymous hemianopia will be present (Fig. 9.6). When the striate cortex of both occipital lobes is affected, usually by an infarct resulting from occlusion of the basilar artery (of which both posterior cerebral arteries are terminal branches), *cortical blindness* results. A characteristic feature of this condition is that the patient may deny or be unaware of their loss of vision (Anton's syndrome). Since the reflex pathways for the pupillary reflexes are not involved, and therefore the pupils react normally to light, the condition can be misdiagnosed as hysterical blindness. Cortical blindness may be a transient phenomenon in migraine, and may follow a relatively minor head injury in children and adolescents.

Papilloedema

Papilloedema refers to oedema of the optic papilla or disc, without reference to its underlying cause. It is commonly caused by raised intracranial pressure.

The optic nerve is a direct extension of the central nervous system. The dura mater fuses with the periosteum of the orbit, and the pia mater and arachnoid mater fuse with the sclera. The optic nerve is therefore surrounded by the subarachnoid space, and a rise in central subarachnoid pressure is freely conducted to the optic subarachnoid space (Fig. 9.7).

Early signs of papilloedema are distension of the veins and blurring of the upper and lower disc margins; the temporal margin is last to become blurred. The next stage is filling in of the physiological cup and elevation of the disc above the retinal levels. Oedema may spread out like a fan across the retina and haemorrhages may appear around the disc. Eventually secondary optic atrophy follows.

Causes of papilloedema include:
(a) Intracranial neoplasms, especially of the posterior fossa or temporal lobe. Papilloedema occurs less commonly in slowly growing tumours when pressure readjustments occur. A tumour near one optic foramen compressing the optic nerve may protect that nerve from raised intracranial pressure; unilateral optic atrophy with papilloedema in the opposite eye results (Foster-Kennedy syndrome).

Fig. 9.7 Pial membranes and subarachnoid space surrounding optic nerve. (Modified from Hayreh, S.S., *Trans. Amer. Acad. Ophthalmol. Otolaryngol.* 1974, **78**: OP241–54.

(b) Abscesses, subdural haematomas, and other space occupying lesions.

(c) Hydrocephalus from any cause including meningitis and sub-arachnoid haemorrhage.

(d) Intracranial venous thrombosis.

(e) Benign intracranial hypertension (see pp. 259–60).

(f) Metabolic disorders, e.g. hypoparathyroidism, emphysema.

(g) Malignant hypertension.

(h) Ischaemic papillopathy from disease of the posterior ciliary artery which supplies the area around the optic disc (Fig. 9.7).

Optic neuritis

Optic neuritis is an inflammation of the optic nerve. If the inflammation is sufficiently anterior to cause swelling of the optic disc, the appearance is described as *papillitis*. If it is situated more posteriorly so that the direct effects of inflammation are not visible ophthalmoscopically it is called *retrobulbar neuritis*. The symptoms of optic neuritis are usually blurring or dimness of vision, and pain in and behind the eye. Examination usually reveals tenderness to pressure of the affected eye, impaired visual acuity, and a central or paracentral scotoma.

The most important and common cause is multiple sclerosis (p. 272); about 50–60% of patients with optic neuritis will eventually develop multiple sclerosis. Other causes include neuromyelitis optica, herpes zoster and other viral infections, meningitis and encephalitis, but in many cases no cause is determined.

Optic atrophy

Optic atrophy is the result of degeneration of optic nerve fibres. Clinically, there is usually impaired visual acuity, a scotoma in the visual field and pallor of the optic disc on ophthalmoscopic examination.

Causes include: compression of optic nerves by tumours, aneurysms; optic neuritis, most commonly in multiple sclerosis; papilloedema, with secondary optic atrophy; toxic causes (e.g. tobacco, lead, alcohol); vitamin deficiencies (e.g. pernicious anaemia); trauma; syphilis; retinal artery occlusion, with secondary optic atrophy; retinal degeneration; hereditary causes (e.g. Leber's optic atrophy and Friedreich's ataxia).

III, IV and VI cranial nerves

The third, fourth and sixth cranial nerves innervate the extraocular muscles. Their chief function is to control ocular movement.

Ocular movements

The ocular movements are carried out by three pairs of muscles: superior and inferior recti; medial and lateral recti; superior and inferior oblique muscles.

In order to understand the function of individual muscles it is necessary to know their planes of action.

The medial and lateral recti move the eye in a horizontal plane, parallel to the floor of the orbit. The superior and inferior recti move the eye in a vertical plane when the eye is turned outwards. If the eye is turned inwards the superior and inferior recti act as rotators of the eye (Fig. 9.8).

The superior and inferior oblique muscles act in a vertical plane when the eye is turned inwards; the superior oblique then acts as a pure depressor and the inferior oblique as an elevator. If the eye is turned outwards the superior and inferior oblique muscles act as rotators of the eye (Fig. 9.8).

From a practical point of view, when testing the actions of the eye muscles, the superior oblique depresses the eye and the inferior oblique elevates it when the eye is turned inwards; the superior rectus elevates

Fig. 9.8 The positions and actions of the superior and inferior rectus muscles, and superior and inferior oblique muscles, in different positions of gaze of the right eye. (Modified from Cogan, 1956.)

and the inferior rectus depresses the eye when it is turned outwards. The actions of the medial and lateral recti are obvious (Fig. 9.9).

The oculomotor (III) nerve innervates the superior rectus, medial rectus, inferior rectus and inferior oblique; the trochlear (IV) nerve supplies the superior oblique; and the abducens (VI) nerve innervates the lateral rectus muscle.

Squint or strabismus

This is the term applied to lack of parallelism of ocular movement. It is important to distinguish between a *paralytic squint* which is caused by weakness or paralysis of an ocular muscle, and a *non-paralytic* or *concomitant* squint which is often congenital and is caused by ocular muscle imbalance.

Paralytic squint   A paralytic squint may become apparent only on eye movement, and is accompanied by double vision (diplopia) in the direction of the gaze of the weakened muscle.

Fig. 9.9 Direction of action of the ocular muscles. (From Lance and McLeod, 1981, with permission of Butterworths, London.)

Non-paralytic squint This is present when both eyes are at rest and is equal for all positions of the eye. If the fixing eye is covered, the movements of the affected eye are full. A non-paralytic squint is usually not associated with diplopia.

Diplopia

Diplopia, or double vision, occurs when there is paresis of one or more ocular muscles. Because the image is projected into the macula of one eye and into another part of the retina of the other, the patient will see two images.

Clinically, the paretic muscle is most easily determined by asking the patient to follow the examiner's finger with the eyes as he moves it in different directions. Cover one eye with a red glass so that the patient may recognize the two images — one white, one red. Find the position of gaze in which the two images are maximally separated. Then (i) the direction in which separation is greatest is the direction of action of the paralysed muscle; (ii) the more peripheral of the two images is the false image and is seen by the affected eye; e.g. if the right lateral rectus muscle is paralysed, the two images will be separated maximally when the eyes are deviated to the right, and the false image will be the one on the extreme right.

III oculomotor nerve

The nucleus of the third nerve lies in the midbrain at the level of the superior colliculus (Figs 9.10, 9.11). It consists of (i) the main oculomotor nucleus, which is the motor nucleus for the medial rectus, superior rectus, inferior rectus, inferior oblique and levator palpebrae superioris muscles, and (ii) Edinger-Westphal nucleus which controls pupillary constriction.

The oculomotor nerve passes through the red nucleus to emerge from the midbrain in the angle between the cerebral peduncles and the pons (Fig. 9.11). It then passes forwards between the posterior cerebral and the superior cerebellar arteries, close to the posterior communicating artery, to enter the cavernous sinus through the dura mater near the posterior clinoid process (Figs 9.10, 9.12, 15.2). It then passes through the cavernous sinus and superior orbital fissure to supply the appropriate extraocular muscles. The nerve to the inferior oblique muscles has a parasympathetic branch which goes to the ciliary ganglion. Sympathetic fibres from the plexus around the internal carotid artery join the first division of the trigeminal nerve in the cavernous sinus.

Fig. 9.10 Origin and course of oculomotor (III) nerve. (Modified from *Grant's Atlas of Anatomy*, 1978, 7th edn, Williams and Wilkins, Baltimore.)

Fig. 9.11 Section of midbrain at the level of superior colliculi.

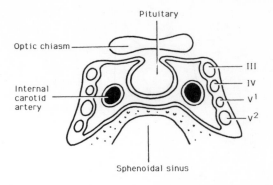

Fig. 9.12 Coronal section of the cavernous sinuses showing the position of cranial nerves in the walls.

Lesions of the third nerve result in varying degrees of paralysis of the muscles which it supplies. A complete lesion of the third nerve results in ptosis, and paralysis of all extraocular muscles except the superior oblique and the lateral rectus. The eye is deviated outwards. The pupil is widely dilated and unreactive.

The third nerve may be affected: (i) in the midbrain, e.g. vascular lesions, glioma. Long tracts are commonly affected as well, causing a contralateral hemiplegia and the brachium conjunctivum may be involved as it passes through the red nucleus causing a cerebellar ataxia and 'red nucleus tremor'; (ii) in its intracranial course, e.g. aneurysms (usually on the posterior communicating artery), meningitis, vascular lesions (diabetes), cavernous sinus thrombosis, tumours; (iii) in the superior orbital fissure (together with the fourth nerve and first division of the fifth nerve) or within the orbit, e.g. inflammatory lesions, tumours, granulomas.

Compressive lesions usually affect the pupilloconstrictor fibres resulting in a dilated pupil, but in a diabetic third nerve palsy the pupil is often spared.

IV trochlear nerve

The trochlear nerve arises from its nucleus at the level of the inferior colliculus in the midbrain. The fibres from the nucleus course dorsally and decussate completely in the roof of the midbrain to emerge behind the inferior colliculi (Fig. 9.13). The nerve then passes anteriorly and ventrally around the cerebral peduncles and enters the cavernous sinus through the dura below the posterior clinoid processes (Fig. 9.12). It enters the orbit through the superior orbital fissure.

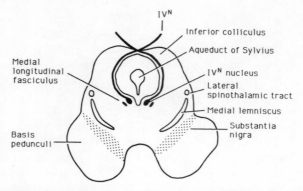

Fig. 9.13 Transverse section of midbrain at level of the inferior colliculi showing the course of the trochlear nerve.

Lesions of the fourth nerve cause paralysis of the superior oblique muscle with extorsion of the eye and weakness of downward gaze. Patients adopt a posture with the head tilted towards the opposite shoulder. The nerve may be involved by conditions similar to those that affect the oculomotor nerve.

VI abducens nerve

The sixth nerve nucleus is situated in the pons beneath the fourth ventricle at the level of the facial colliculus (Fig. 9.14). Fibres leave the

Fig. 9.14 Section of pons showing course of abducens (VI) and facial (VII) nerves.

nucleus and course anteriorly through the tegmentum of the pons to emerge from the brainstem at the lower border of the pons (Fig. 15.2). The nerve then passes forwards and laterally over the tip of the petrous temporal bone, pierces the dura mater alongside the dorsum sellae and enters the cavernous sinus (Fig. 9.12). It subsequently enters the orbit through the superior orbital fissure.

Lesions of the sixth nerve result in paralysis of abduction of the eye and may be due to causes similar to those which produce lesions of the third and fourth nerves. Because of its long intracranial course, the sixth nerve is often involved secondarily to raised intracranial pressure; the pressure results in the nerve being stretched as it passes over the tip of the petrous temporal bone. Infection of the petrous temporal bone, resulting from chronic middle ear infection, may involve the sixth nerve and the first division of the fifth nerve (Gradenigo's syndrome, p. 292). This is an example of a 'false localizing sign', since the sixth nerve palsy is not the result of a primary lesion of the nerve.

Conjugate movements of the eyes

Saccadic movements of the eyes rapidly fixate the image of a new object on the macula; *pursuit* movements are slower and enable the image of a moving target to remain on the macula. Saccadic movements are generated through the pathway from the frontal eye fields to the paramedian pontine reticular formation (PPRF) for horizontal conjugate gaze, and to the midbrain for vertical gaze. Pursuit movements are controlled by pathways from the occipital areas (Figs 9.15, 9.16).

The *medial longitudinal fasciculus* is a fibre tract that runs in the brainstem in close relationship to the third, fourth and sixth nerve nuclei (Fig. 9.15). It coordinates the actions of the nerves to the extraocular muscles with each other and with the vestibular apparatus (thus maintaining visual fixation during rapid head movements — vestibulo-ocular reflexes), and it relays impulses for horizontal conjugate gaze from the PPRF to the medial rectus muscles.

Control of horizontal conjugate deviation of the eyes (Fig. 9.15).

The following regions of the brain are involved in the control of horizontal conjugate gaze.

Frontal   Voluntary eye movements are initiated from the frontal eye fields (area 8) at the posterior end of the second frontal convolution. Corticofugal fibres pass through the internal capsule and course

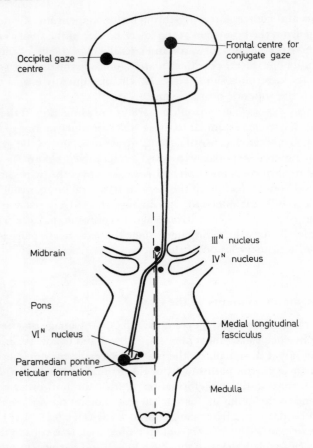

Fig. 9.15 Pathways for horizontal eye movements. (From Lance and McLeod, 1981, with permission of Butterworths, London.)

downwards to decussate at the rostral end of the midbrain and terminate in the PPRF, near the sixth nerve nucleus.

Occipital A centre for conjugate eye movements also exists in the occipital region, since conjugate deviation can be produced by stimulation of areas 17, 18, and 19. This is concerned with tracking (pursuit) movements of the eyes in response to visual stimuli.

Pontine centre There is a pontine centre for horizontal conjugate gaze situated in the region of the sixth nucleus (PPRF).

Fig. 9.16 Pathways for vertical eye movements. (From Lance and McLeod, 1981, with permission of Butterworths, London.)

Control of vertical conjugate deviation (Fig. 9.16).

The following regions of the brain are involved in vertical conjugate gaze: (a) Cortical centre in the frontal and occipital lobes which are the same as those for horizontal gaze. Descending pathways decussate above the level of the superior colliculi. (b) A midbrain centre at the level of the superior colliculi.

Lesions resulting in gaze palsies

Horizontal gaze palsies   In considering disorders of ocular movements it is of great clinical importance to distinguish supranuclear lesions (which do not cause diplopia because both eyes continue to move along parallel axes) from nuclear and infranuclear lesions which do cause diplopia.

(a) Cerebral — *Irritative* lesions of the frontal region, and sometimes of the occipital region, may result in turning of the head and eyes to the side opposite the lesion, e.g. in focal epilepsy (versive seizures). *Paralytic* lesions, such as occur after strokes and injuries, cause a deviation of the eyes to the side of the lesion because of the unopposed stimulus arising from the opposite cortex.

(b) Basal ganglia — *Irritative* lesions are seen in postencephalitic Parkinsonism and give rise to oculogyric crises. *Paralytic* lesions may also be seen in Parkinson's disease causing fixity of gaze and rigidity of eye movements.

(c) Pons — Pontine lesions (e.g. vascular and demyelinating disorders, encephalitis, gliomas, Wernicke's encephalopathy) may cause impairment of conjugate deviation to the side of the lesion. Usually this is accompanied by nystagmus, and involvement of neighbouring cranial nerves, nuclei and long tracts.

Vertical gaze palsies　(a) Cerebral — Cerebral lesions, especially if irritative, may cause impairment of vertical as well as horizontal conjugate gaze, but the vertical component is relatively insignificant.

(b) Tectum — *Irritative* lesions may cause oculogyric crises. *Paralytic* lesions usually are in the region of the superior colliculus.

Parinaud's syndrome is caused by a lesion in the tectum, e.g. a pinealoma, and consists of paralysis of vertical eye movements, impaired vergence, and pupils that do not react to light but may continue to react to accommodation. Unlike Argyll Robertson pupils, they are not constricted or irregular.

Paralysis of upward gaze may also be found with lesions of the fourth ventricle and cerebellum due to upward transtentorial herniation, but it is not associated with pupillary abnormalities. Loss of voluntary vertical eye movements, particularly down gaze, with retention of reflex movement is characteristic of progressive supranuclear palsy (Steel-Richardson syndrome).

Paralysis of vergence　Impairment of vergence has been reported with occipital lesions but is most commonly seen with lesions of the midbrain in the region of the superior colliculus.

Internuclear ophthalmoplegia　An important disorder of eye movement is caused by a lesion of the medial longitudinal fasciculus. It is characterized by weakness of adduction of one eye on conjugate lateral deviation,

Right   Left

Fig. 9.17 Internuclear ophthalmoplegia. The left eye does not adduct (lesion of the left medial longitudinal fasciculus) and there is nystagmus in the abducting right eye.

associated with nystagmus in the opposite (abducting) eye (Fig. 9.17). It may be bilateral or unilateral. If lesions are caudally placed, near the sixth nerve nucleus, vergence is intact. With more rostrally placed lesions, near the third nerve nucleus, vergence may be affected. Bilateral internuclear ophthalmoplegia is usually caused by multiple sclerosis, but the unilateral condition more often results from vascular lesions. Mild forms may be detected by observing the visual axes during saccadic movements as the examiner asks the patient to fix the eyes alternately on one finger, then the other.

Nystagmus

Nystagmus is a disorder of eye movements characterized by involuntary rhythmic oscillations. The eyes normally remain stationary if the tone of the muscles is equal and opposite in all directions. The tone of the ocular muscles depends upon innervation derived from various sources, e.g. cerebral, brainstem, labyrinthine, ocular and cervical cord (neck muscles). Any interruption of these pathways may cause alteration in tone giving rise to an unsteadiness of the posture of the eyes, which is manifested as nystagmus.

Nystagmus may be *pendular* (oscillating) or *jerk* (rhythmic).

Pendular nystagmus

This is characterized by oscillations that are approximately equal in rate for the two directions of movement. It is due to loss of central vision and of the normal reflex tonic innervation from the retina. It is observed in those who have lost vision early in life, and in people who have worked in poor light for many years (miner's nystagmus). Some cases are congenital.

Jerk nystagmus

The oscillations are faster in one direction than the other and the direction of the nystagmus is designated by the direction of the fast component. Nystagmus may be horizontal, vertical or rotatory.

Opsoclonus is the term applied to rapid multidirectional eye movements usually associated with severe brain disease.

Oscillopsia is the visual sensation of movement of the environment experienced by subjects with nystagmus.

Causes of jerk nystagmus

(a) Opticokinetic nystagmus. This is a normal phenomenon when the eyes are following a series of objects moving across the field of vision, e.g. looking out of a train window. The slow phase represents the normal pursuit movement of the eyes, and the fast phase represents the corrective movement which brings the eyes back to the central position (saccadic movement). Opticokinetic responses can be elicited clinically with a rotating drum marked with vertical stripes and may be helpful in determining the site of a lesion causing hemianopia. The opticokinetic responses remain normal in lesions of the optic tract; an impairment of opticokinetic responses occurs with a cerebral lesion. With unilateral cerebral lesions (with or without hemianopia), particularly those in the parieto-occipital region, the opticokinetic responses will be disturbed when the stimulus moves towards the site of the lesion.

(b) Vestibular nystagmus. Each vestibular system is responsible for exerting a tonic effect causing drift of the eyes to the opposite side. Normally vestibular effects are balanced so that the eyes are stable. Damage to the vestibular system causes an imbalance, requiring a fast corrective movement to the side opposite the lesion (jerk nystagmus). This type of nystagmus is seen normally during rotation (the slow component is opposite to the direction of rotation). Clinically, vestibular nystagmus is seen in disease of the labyrinth or vestibular nerve (e.g. labyrinthitis, Menière's disease, vestibular neuronitis) or their connections in the brainstem (e.g. multiple sclerosis, vascular lesions, encephalitis). The fast component is directed towards the side of the lesion.

Vertical nystagmus is nearly always the result of a lesion of the central nervous system, usually in the brainstem. It almost never occurs in lesions of the labyrinth or vestibular nerve.

(c) Nystagmus in cerebellar lesions. Nystagmus is common in disorders affecting the cerebellum, particularly if its connections with the vestibular nuclei are involved. The fast component of cerebellar nystagmus is directed towards the side of the lesion.

(d) Nystagmus from weakness of ocular movements. Nystagmus may occur where there is weakness of conjugate lateral gaze. This can occur in normal individuals at extremes of ocular deviation, in fatigue, myasthenia, and in cerebral lesions which affect conjugate gaze (frontal, occipital, brainstem).

(e) Congenital nystagmus. Congenital nystagmus may be either pendular or jerk, and may be inherited.

(f) Cervical cord lesions. Lesions of the upper cervical cord may occasionally cause nystagmus because of interruption of the pathways subserving the tonic neck reflexes.

The pupils

In examining the pupils one should note their size, equality, regularity, and reaction to light and accommodation. The size of the pupil depends upon the reciprocal actions of the sphincter muscle, which is innervated by the parasympathetic nerves, and the dilator muscle, which is innervated by the sympathetic nerves (Fig. 9.18).

The *sympathetic pupillodilator fibres* arise in the hypothalamus, descend in the lateral tegmentum of the midbrain, pons and medulla to synapse on cells of the intermediolateral column at C8, T1, T2.

Preganglionic sympathetic fibres leave the cervical cord at this level and course through the ventral roots and white rami to the superior cervical ganglion where they synapse.

Postganglionic fibres travel from the superior cervical ganglion along the common carotid artery to its bifurcation. Most fibres responsible for

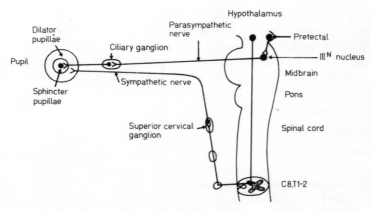

Fig. 9.18 Innervation of the pupil. (From Lance and McLeod, 1981, with permission of Butterworths, London.)

sweating and vasomotor function of the face travel with the external carotid artery, but those responsible for sweating on the medial aspect of the forehead, and the pupillodilator fibres, travel with the internal carotid artery to the carotid siphon. At the petrous temporal bone, and at the cavernous sinus, the sympathetic pupillodilator fibres join and course with the first division of the trigeminal nerve.

The *parasympathetic pupilloconstrictor fibres* arise in the Edinger-Westphal nucleus and course in the third nerve to the ciliary ganglion where they synapse. The postganglionic fibres emerge as the ciliary nerves.

The light reflex

The afferent pathway of the light reflex is from the retina, along the optic nerve to the optic tract where the fibres part from those which are destined for the lateral geniculate body and instead go to the pretectal region. There is a pathway from the pretectal region to the third nucleus of both sides, thus accounting for direct and consensual light reflexes. The efferent pathway is in the third nerve (Fig. 9.19).

In a lesion of the third nerve, the pupil will be dilated. The direct light reaction, and the consensual response elicited by shining a light in the other eye, will be absent. However, the consensual reaction of the unaffected eye will be present when a light is shone in the affected eye.

In blindness due to optic radiation or cortical lesions (but not optic nerve or tract lesions), both direct and consensual reflexes of both eyes will be present.

Accommodation reflex

The accommodation reflex is associated with convergence of the eyes ('near response'). The descending pathways project from the parieto-occipital cortex to the midbrain (Edinger-Westphal nucleus).

Any lesion involving the pupilloconstrictor fibres will impair the reaction of accommodation. Selective impairment of accommodation may occur in some midbrain lesions.

Argyll Robertson pupil

Douglas Argyll Robertson, an Edinburgh physician, described pupils that are small, irregular, unequal, dilate poorly with mydriatics and react to accommodation but not to light. They are observed most commonly in syphilis, but also occasionally in some other disorders, e.g. diabetes. The site of the lesion is uncertain but is probably in the pretectal region.

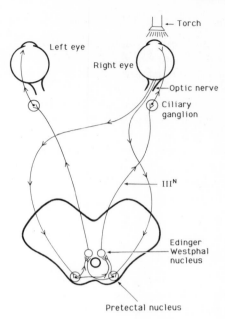

Fig. 9.19 Pathways of the pupillary light reflex for direct and consensual responses. (Modified from Duke-Elder and Scott, *System of Ophthalmology*, **XII**, 1971, Kimpton, London.)

Pseudo-Argyll Robertson pupils may occur in midbrain lesions. They do not react to light, but they are neither small nor irregular.

Adie's pupil (tonic pupil of Adie; Holmes-Adie syndrome)

This condition occurs mainly in females and the onset is usually sudden with the complaint of blurred vision. One pupil is larger than the other, but the pupillary abnormality is bilateral in 20% of cases. The pupil reacts very sluggishly to light and accommodation, and will pass slowly through the full range of constriction. On relaxation, dilatation proceeds slowly. Knee and ankle jerks may be absent and the syndrome must therefore be distinguished from tabes dorsalis which it superficially resembles. The instillation of 2.5% methacholine eye-drops causes Adie's pupil, but not the normal pupil, to constrict. On slit-lamp examination, the margin of the iris may be seen to undulate.

Pathological changes have been demonstrated in the ciliary ganglion. Synaptic transmission is impaired in the spinal monosynaptic reflex arc, accounting for the absent reflexes.

Horner's syndrome

Horner's syndrome results from a lesion of oculosympathetic fibres anywhere along their pathway, e.g. brainstem, cervical cord, first thoracic root, cervical sympathetic trunk or intracranial course (Fig. 9.18).

The characteristic features are: ptosis (sympathetic fibres supply the smooth muscle of upper eyelids); pupillary constriction; enophthalmos; and anhidrosis of one side of the face, if the lesion is proximal to the carotid bifurcation (since sympathetic fibres to the face course with the external carotid artery) or of the medial side of the forehead if the lesion is distal to the bifurcation. It should be noted that the ptosis in Horner's syndrome is only partial and never complete as it is in a third nerve palsy.

V trigeminal nerve

The fifth nerve contains motor and sensory fibres. It arises from the lateral aspect of the inferior surface of the pons (Fig. 15.2) by two roots, a large sensory and a small motor root. The roots pierce the dura mater to join the trigeminal or Gasserian ganglion which lies between two layers of dura mater on the apex of the petrous temporal bone.

The *sensory root*, the ganglion cells of which lie in the Gasserian ganglion, has three main divisions:

(a) Ophthalmic, which passes through the lateral wall of the cavernous sinus to enter the orbit through the superior orbital fissure (Fig. 9.12). It supplies sensation to the nose, forehead, scalp and upper lid as well as to the cornea and the mucous membrane of the frontal sinuses (Fig. 9.20). Dura mater of the falx and superior surface of the tentorium is supplied by the tentorial nerve arising from the ophthalmic division.

(b) Maxillary, which courses through the foramen rotundum into the pterygopalatine fossa and then enters the orbit through the inferior orbital fissure. It leaves the orbit as the infra-orbital nerve. It supplies the skin of the lower lid, alae nasae, the upper lip and a 2–3 cm strip on the face, anterior to a line which extends from the outer angle of the mouth through a point midway between the outer canthus of the eye and the ear (Fig. 9.20).

(c) Mandibular, which leaves with the motor root through the foramen ovale. It supplies the skin of the lower jaw, part of the face, and lateral aspect of the ear and the external auditory meatus (Fig. 9.20); it also innervates the mucous membrane of the cheek, the anterior two-thirds of the tongue, and the floor of the mouth. Meningeal branches supply the dura mater above the tentorium.

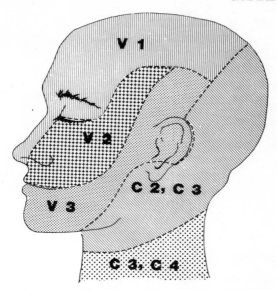

Fig. 9.20 Cutaneous innervation of the face. (Modified from Brodal, 1969, *Neurological Anatomy in Relation to Clinical Medicine*, 2nd edn, Oxford University Press, Oxford.)

The *motor root* innervates the temporalis muscle, the masseter, pterygoids, anterior belly of the digastric, mylohyoid, tensor tympani and tensor palati muscles.

Central connections of the fifth nerve

The *sensory nucleus* is in three parts (Fig. 9.21).

(a) The main sensory nucleus, which is in the lateral part of the pons, receives the sensory fibres concerned with tactile and postural sensibility; second order neurones cross to the quintothalamic tracts, near the medial lemniscus.

(b) The nucleus of the spinal tract extends downwards in the lateral part of the medulla to about the level of C2 where it is continuous with the substantia gelatinosa. It receives the pain and temperature fibres from the fifth nerve. The ophthalmic division terminates in the more caudal part, and the mandibular division terminates in the most cephalic part of the nucleus. Second order neurones cross to the quintothalamic tracts.

(c) The mesencephalic nucleus lies cephalad to the main sensory nucleus and receives the muscle afferent fibres which run in the motor root.

Fig. 9.21 Nuclei and fibre tracts in the brainstem of the trigeminal nerve.
(Modified from Brodal, 1965, *The Cranial Nerves. Anatomy and anatomico-clinical correlations*, 2nd edn, Blackwell Scientific Publications, Oxford.)

The *motor nucleus* is situated in the mid-pons, medially to the main sensory nucleus.

Lesions of the fifth nerve

Central lesions of the fifth nerve in the brainstem are usually associated with palsies of other cranial nerves and involvement of long tracts. A lesion in the pons may cause loss of tactile sensation over the trigeminal nerve distribution with preservation of painful sensation which is relayed in the spinal tract. A lesion in the medulla, [e.g. syringobulbia, posterior inferior cerebellar artery thrombosis (PICA syndrome)] may cause loss of pain and temperature sensation (spinal tract of V), but preservation of light touch (main sensory nucleus in pons). Peripheral lesions may give rise to pain, paraesthesiae, and sensory loss over the distribution of the trigeminal nerve. Such lesions may result from a tumour of the fifth nerve, herpes zoster, or compression by adjacent tumours (e.g. meningioma, acoustic neuroma).

Trigeminal neuralgia (see pp. 302–3)

This is a distressing disorder, characterized by *paroxysmal brief* attacks of severe pain in the distribution of the fifth nerve, usually in its second and third divisions. The condition affects usually, but not exclusively, middle-aged people. The pain is burning and jabbing, and it tends to be precipitated by chewing, cold, talking, swallowing, or touching 'trigger zones'. There are no sensory abnormalities detectable on neurological examination. The probable causes include spontaneous repetitive discharges from the Gasserian ganglion or spinal nucleus of the fifth nerve, or pressure on roots by tumours or small arteries.

The pain of trigeminal neuralgia, or *tic douloureux* has to be differentiated from constant, dull facial pain due to: pressure on the fifth nerve; pain arising in sinuses, teeth, eyes (glaucoma) and temporomandibular joints; or atypical facial neuralgia.

VII facial nerve

The seventh cranial nerve consists of two parts: the *facial nerve* which innervates the muscles of facial expression, together with the stapedius muscle, stylohyoid and posterior belly of the digastric; and the *nervus intermedius*, which carries taste fibres from the anterior two-thirds of the tongue and parasympathetic secretory fibres to the lacrimal, submandibular and sublingual glands.

Facial nerve

The nucleus of the facial nerve is situated caudally in the lateral part of the pons. The emerging fibres pass backwards to form a loop around the sixth nerve nucleus, before passing ventrolaterally to emerge from the lateral aspect of the caudal part of the pons (Fig. 9.14). Together with the eighth nerve and nervus intermedius it enters the internal auditory meatus and courses laterally in the facial canal of the petrous temporal bone. It turns sharply backwards on the medial aspect of the middle ear to form the genu, where the geniculate ganglion is situated, and then downwards to emerge from the skull at the stylomastoid foramen (Fig. 9.22). It pierces the parotid gland and divides into branches which supply the muscles of the face as well as the stylohyoid and posterior belly of digastric muscles.

Supranuclear fibres are derived from (a) corticobulbar tracts, which arise mainly from area 4, and which are crossed. However, the upper part of the facial musculature receives a bilateral upper motor neurone innervation; and (b) extrapyramidal fibres, which are concerned with emotional expression.

Fig. 9.22 The facial nerve. (Modified from Walton, 1977, *Brain's Diseases of the Nervous System*, 8th edn, Oxford University Press, Oxford.)

Nervus intermedius

Efferent fibres originate from the cells of the superior salivary nucleus close to the facial nucleus. Those destined for the lacrimal gland leave the nervus intermedius near the geniculate ganglion in the greater superficial petrosal nerve (Fig. 9.22). Those destined for the sublingual and submaxillary glands travel in the chorda tympani.

Afferent fibres, which convey taste from the anterior two-thirds of the tongue and travel in the lingual and chorda tympani nerves, have their cell nuclei in the geniculate ganglion. They terminate centrally in the nucleus of the tractus solitarius.

Lesions of the facial nerve

It is important clinically to distinguish between upper and lower motor neurone lesions.

Upper motor neurone lesions of the face are commonly seen in strokes in which there is a capsular haemorrhage or infarction. As well as a hemiplegia of the opposite side there is weakness of the facial musculature. This is usually noted as asymmetry, with drooping of the angle of the mouth and loss of the nasolabial fold. The upper part of the face — frontalis and the orbicularis oculi muscles — is nearly always involved to a lesser extent than the lower part of the face because of the bilateral corticobulbar innervation of the relevant part of the facial nucleus. Facial movements in response to emotional reactions are often normal, even though voluntary movements are impaired, since emotional expression is mediated through frontopontine pathways. Sometimes, the upper and lower face are equally affected and then the facial palsy can be distinguished clinically from a lower motor neurone paralysis by the retention of emotional expression.

Lower motor neurone lesions of the face are most commonly seen in *Bell's palsy*. This is a relatively common condition of uncertain aetiology, characterized by sudden onset of facial weakness or paralysis. The upper and lower facial muscles are equally affected, and are paralysed for both voluntary and involuntary movements. The patient cannot close the eye, pout, or whistle, and the angle of the mouth droops.

If the lesion is proximal to the level of separation of the chorda tympani, taste over the anterior two-thirds of the tongue will be lost. If the lesion lies proximal to the greater superficial petrosal nerve, lacrimation will also be impaired (Fig. 9.22). If the nerve to stapedius is involved, there will be hyperacusis, i.e. an intensification of loud noises.

Facial palsies may also occur in: pontine lesions, when they are usually accompanied by lateral rectus palsy and long tract signs; peripheral neuropathies; fractures of the petrous temporal bone; middle ear infections; geniculate herpes; acoustic neuromas or other tumours.

VIII acoustic nerve

The eighth nerve contains two groups of fibres — those in the cochlear branch, which are concerned with hearing, and those in the vestibular branch which are concerned with posture and equilibrium.

The cochlear nerve

The peripheral processes of the cochlear nerve are in contact with the cells of the spiral organ of Corti in the inner ear. The cell bodies lie in the spiral ganglion, and the central processes pass with the eighth nerve through the internal auditory meatus to enter the brainstem at the lower border of the pons, where they synapse in the cochlear nucleus. Fibres cross in the trapezoid body, synapse in the superior olivary complex of nuclei, and pass rostrally in the lateral lemniscus to the medial geniculate body and inferior colliculus, and thence to the auditory cortex in the superior temporal gyrus. Hearing is bilaterally represented in the cerebral cortex.

The major symptoms of disease of the cochlear nerve are tinnitus (a sensation of noise or ringing in the ears, usually a whistling or hissing sound) and deafness. The clinical examination of hearing is described in Chapter 2.

Audiometric testing (measuring of hearing threshold at various frequencies) enables more accurate assessment of auditory function to be made and should always be performed when hearing loss is suspected from the application of tests described above. Specialized audiometric tests, such as loudness recruitment and tone decay, help to localize the lesion causing deafness to cochlea, nerve or brainstem.

Causes of nerve deafness

Endorgan — Noise; old age; drugs, e.g. aminoglycosides, diuretics; congenital and hereditary causes; trauma; Menière's disease.
Nerve — cerebellopontine angle tumour; vascular lesions; trauma; hereditary causes.

Cortical deafness is very rare and requires the presence of bilateral lesions in the superior temporal gyrus.

Vestibular nerve

The vestibular branch of the eighth nerve is concerned with the maintenance of posture and balance. It receives afferent impulses from the utricle, saccule and semicircular canals in the labyrinth (Fig. 9.23). There are three semicircular canals on each side — an anterior vertical, a posterior vertical and a horizontal canal — which are arranged in planes at right angles to one another. The posterior vertical canal is in a vertical plane parallel to that of the anterior vertical canal of the other side. When the head is inclined 30° forwards from the vertical, the lateral canals are horizontal. The semicircular canals respond to angular acceleration.

On the other hand, the otolith organs in the utricle and saccule signal the static position of the head in space and respond to linear acceleration (Fig. 9.23).

The vestibular nerve has its cell bodies in the vestibular ganglion of

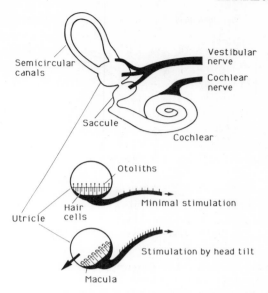

Fig. 9.23 Schema of the internal ear showing a stylized version of the otolith organ in the utricle. When the head is in such a position that otoliths hang from hair cells, labyrinthine stimulation is maximal, as indicated by the vertical strokes (representing nerve impulses) superimposed on the branch of the vestibular nerve. (From Lance and McLeod, 1981, with permission of Butterworths, London.)

Scarpa in the internal auditory meatus. The central processes pass with the cochlear nerve to the lower border of the pons. There the cochlear and vestibular nerves part company, the vestibular nerve passing more medially to terminate in the vestibular nuclei. The vestibular nuclei have four main parts and are connected to: the anterior horn cells of the spinal cord by the vestibulospinal tract; the ocular motor neurones by the medial longitudinal fasciculus; the flocculonodular lobe of the cerebellum; and the reticular formation (Fig. 9.24).

Examination of the vestibular function of the eighth nerve

Disorders of the vestibular branch of the eighth nerve may be manifested by nystagmus, disturbance of gait, balance and muscular control. There are two special tests of vestibular function that are of particular importance.

Caloric tests   The patient lies on a couch, face up, with the neck flexed 30° to the horizontal plane and eyes looking straight ahead. In this position

Fig. 9.24 Some anatomical connections of the vestibular nuclei. Fibres ascending to the nuclei responsible for eye movement in the median longitudinal fasciculus take origin from all four of the large vestibular nuclei, and descending fibres from the medial nucleus only. The vestibulospinal tract arises from the lateral vestibular nucleus in which cells are arranged somatotopically, thus permitting the effects of cerebellovestibular connections (not shown) to be distributed to localized areas of the spinal cord. (From Lance and McLeod, 1981, with permission of Butterworths, London.)

the horizontal canals are vertical. Water at 30°C is run into one ear for 40 s and the duration and slow phase velocity of nystagmus (fast component to opposite side with cold water) is measured. The opposite ear is then similarly irrigated and the same measurements made. The procedure is then repeated with water of temperature 44°C which in normal subjects induces nystagmus beating to the same side as the irrigation.

Two major types of abnormality may be observed:

(a) Canal paresis. This term indicates an absence of response to caloric irrigation of one ear and occurs with peripheral lesions, e.g. labyrinthitis, vestibular neuronitis, Menière's disease, acoustic neuroma.

(b) Directional preponderance. This is a term used to describe the unmasking of latent imbalance of tonic vestibular mechanisms. Cold water in the left ear and warm water in the right ear both cause nystagmus to the right. If these reactions are more pronounced than corresponding reactions producing nystagmus to the left there is said to be a right directional preponderance. It occurs mainly with brainstem lesions but also can be present in peripheral lesions. The directional preponderance can be interpreted as a latent nystagmus to that side and is therefore toward the side of a cerebellar lesion but away from the side of a vestibular lesion.

Combined responses, i.e. canal paresis with directional preponderance, may also occur.

Nystagmus is usually recorded electrically by electronystagmography (ENG) which allows nystagmus to be recorded in darkness. In labyrinthine lesions nystagmus is exaggerated in darkness, by eliminating visual function, but this is not the case in brainstem lesions.

Positional tests Disease or damage to the otolith organ (e.g. trauma, vascular disease, infection) may result in giddiness and nystagmus on sudden head movements. The condition is known as positional nystagmus or vertigo.

In order to test for positional nystagmus the patient sits on a couch, and the head is held and rotated horizontally 30–40° by the observer. The patient is then briskly laid back over the end of the couch so that the head is 30° below horizontal. In normal people, there is no nystagmus. In positional nystagmus, rotatory nystagmus towards the lowermost ear (if this is the affected one) will develop after a latent interval and will fatigue in less than a minute. On sitting up again, nystagmus may recur. In brainstem and cerebellar lesions, there is no latent interval and the nystagmus continues without fatiguing.

Vertigo

Vertigo may be defined as an abnormal perception of movement of the body in relation to the environment, or of apparent movement of the surroundings in relation to the body. There is usually a sense of turning either of the person, or of the outside world. However, the patient may complain of a rocking movement, or of a tendency to veer to one side when walking, or that the outside world tends to move towards or away from him or her.

Vertigo is the commonest symptom of labyrinthine disorders, but does not occur exclusively in these conditions.

The maintenance of equilibrium and posture and the awareness of the position of the body in space depend upon visual impulses from the retina, labyrinthine impulses, and proprioceptive impulses from joints and muscles of the neck, trunk and limbs. Disturbances of equilibrium may therefore have origins other than disease of labyrinthine pathways.

It is very important to obtain a careful history from patients who complain of disorders of equilibrium. Patients may say they suffer from 'dizziness' or 'giddiness', but it cannot be regarded as true vertigo unless there is some sense of rotation or movement of the environment. True vertigo is often accompanied by nausea or vomiting. Dizziness or giddiness in many cases may really be a feeling of light-headedness or faintness or weakness, and not a true disturbance of equilibrium. It is essential to find out what sensation the patients actually experience during their attacks, and to realize that their definitions of dizziness and giddiness may be different from those used in medical practice.

Causes of vertigo

Cortical disturbances   Vertigo may occur as an aura of an epileptic seizure arising in one temporal lobe, or a symptom of migraine and cerebral tumours.

Ocular disturbances   Vertigo may be experienced by some people on looking down from heights, or when ocular palsies result in double vision; or it may accompany opticokinetic nystagmus when a subject looks at fast-moving objects.

Cerebellar disturbances   Vertigo occurs particularly if the vestibular connections with the flocculonodular lobe are involved (Fig. 10.3).

Brainstem lesions   Lesions of the brainstem (e.g. vascular lesions) and multiple sclerosis can cause a severe and prolonged vertigo associated with nystagmus. Brainstem lesions should be suspected if vertigo is prolonged for several weeks, there is no associated deafness or tinnitus, there is vertical nystagmus, brainstem nuclei or tracts are involved, there is directional preponderance without canal paresis on caloric testing, or electronystagmography shows that nystagmus does not become more pronounced when the eyes are closed, in contrast to vestibular nystagmus.

Lesions of the vestibular nerve and labyrinth

(a) Labyrinthine (aural) vertigo. This tends to occur in acute attacks, lasting for only 1–2 h. Often there is associated tinnitus and deafness. Causes include: drugs, e.g. quinine, aminoglycosides; vascular lesions of labyrinth; acute labyrinthitis; motion sickness; and Menière's disease. *Menière's disease* is a condition in which recurrent attacks of severe vertigo are associated with tinnitus and deafness. It is commonly unilateral and is usually a benign and self-limiting condition, but runs a protracted course. It occurs mainly in middle age, and the pathology is a degeneration of the organ of Corti with dilatation of the endolymph system. There is an end-organ (cochlear) deafness and a canal paresis on caloric testing.

(b) Lesions of the eighth nerve. (i) Vertigo is rarely caused by cerebellopontine angle tumours, or meningeal inflammation involving the eighth nerve directly. Deafness and tinnitus are associated. (ii) Vestibular neuronitis (epidemic vertigo). Severe, prostrating vertigo usually starts suddenly, without associated deafness or tinnitus, lasting for days or even a few weeks, and accompanied by nausea and vomiting. There may be a preceding viral infection. Caloric testing usually demonstrates a canal paresis, but there may be a directional preponderance. (iii) Drugs. Ototoxic drugs (e.g. aminoglycosides and salicylates) may cause vertigo. Dizziness and sense of disequilibrium can be caused by many drugs including alcohol, anticonvulsants and sedatives. (iv) Benign recurrent vertigo. This condition is often confused with Menière's disease. The cause is uncertain but it is thought to be a periodic syndrome allied to migraine.

IX glossopharyngeal nerve

The glossopharyngeal nerve arises from a series of rootlets on the lateral surface of the medulla and courses with nerves X and XI through the jugular foramen (Fig. 9.25). It lies in the neck in association with the carotid vessels and jugular vein. It contains motor fibres which arise from the nucleus ambiguus, and innervate the stylopharyngeus muscle. Afferent fibres which run in the glossopharyngeal nerve have their cell bodies in the petrosal ganglion of the nerve. Peripheral branches carry sensory impulses from the posterior third of the tongue, tonsils, soft palate, and posterior wall of the pharynx; centrally directed fibres terminate in the nucleus of the tractus solitarius. A tympanic branch transmits sensation from the tympanic cavity. Secretory fibres arise in the inferior salivatory nucleus and travel to the parotid gland (Fig. 9.25).

Together with the vagus nerve and central part of the accessory nerve, the glossopharyngeal nerve is examined clinically by means of the gag reflex, and by testing palatal and pharyngeal sensation.

The glossopharyngeal nerve is very rarely involved in isolation. In association with the vagus and accessory nerves it may be compressed by tumours of the posterior fossa in the jugular foramen or in the upper part of the neck.

Glossopharyngeal neuralgia has characteristics similar to those of trigeminal neuralgia. Intense paroxysmal pain of brief duration is exper-

Fig. 9.25 The glossopharyngeal nerve. (Modified from *Grant's Atlas of Anatomy*, 1978, 7th edn, Williams and Wilkins, Baltimore.)

ienced in the side of the throat and may radiate to the ear because the sensory part of the vagus nerve is usually implicated in the discharge. Attacks may be precipitated by swallowing.

X vagus nerve

The vagus nerve contains both motor and sensory fibres (Fig. 9.26). It leaves the medulla and passes through the jugular foramen to enter the carotid sheath with nerves IX and XI.

Motor fibres are derived from the nucleus ambiguus in the medulla, whence fibres travel in the vagus to supply the muscles of the palate, pharynx and larynx. General visceral efferents also run in the vagus to the parasympathetic ganglia of the vagal plexuses that innervate the

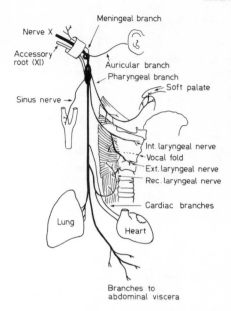

Fig. 9.26 The vagus nerve. (Modified from *Grant's Atlas of Anatomy,* 1978, 7th edn, Williams and Wilkins, Baltimore.)

thoracic and abdominal viscera. They have their cell bodies in the dorsal nucleus of the vagus beneath the floor of the fourth ventricle.

Sensory fibres supply the dura mater of the posterior fossa and part of the ear and external auditory meatus and terminate centrally in the sensory nucleus of the fifth nerve. Fibres supplying sensation to larynx, trachea, oesophagus, thoracic and abdominal viscera terminate centrally in the nucleus of the tractus solitarius.

Lesions of the vagus nerve

Paralysis of the palate

This will result from lesions involving the nucleus ambiguus or the vagus above its pharyngeal branch.

A unilateral paralysis causes few symptoms, but on examination the palate does not fully elevate on the affected side and the uvula is drawn to the unaffected side.

With bilateral palatal palsies, fluids and food regurgitate into the back of the nose on swallowing and speech takes on a nasal quality; words are characteristically mispronounced, e.g. 'eng' instead of 'egg'.

Paralysis of the pharynx

There may be no symptoms from a unilateral lesion, but with a bilateral lesion swallowing becomes difficult, and the pharyngeal reflex is lost.

Paralysis of the larynx

Unilateral paralysis will result from a lesion of the recurrent laryngeal nerve. There may be no symptoms, but usually the voice is hoarse. The affected cord will be seen to lie near the midline. Unilateral paralysis will also result from lesions above the nodose ganglion, but there will be an associated paralysis of the palate and pharynx.

Bilateral paralysis of the larynx results in hoarse voice, difficulty in coughing, and respiratory stridor.

Visceral effects of vagal injury

These are rarely conspicuous clinically. A tachycardia may follow bilateral vagal injury, e.g. polyneuritis.

Causes of vagus nerve lesions   (i) Nuclear lesions in the medulla may result from poliomyelitis, motor neurone disease, diphtheria, syringobulbia, or vascular occlusions. (ii) Posterior fossa tumours, which usually also involve nerves IX, XI and XII. (iii) The main trunk of the vagus in the neck may be damaged by tumours or trauma. If the lesion lies above the superior laryngeal nerve there will be anaesthesia of one side of the larynx, with total ipsilateral vocal cord paralysis. (iv) The recurrent laryngeal nerve may be involved by lymphadenopathies or carcinoma in the neck or thorax, or on the left side by an aortic aneurysm. It may also be affected by a mononeuritis of viral or immune origin. There will be unilateral cord paralysis, but no sensory loss.

XI accessory nerve

The central accessory nerve is functionally part of the vagus nerve and supplies motor fibres to the palate and pharynx.

The spinal accessory nerve is purely motor and supplies the sternomastoid and trapezius muscles through its spinal branch, which arises from C1–5 segments, ascends through the foramen magnum and leaves the skull through the jugular foramen. It may be involved by tumours in the posterior fossa or at its exit from the skull, or in its peripheral course behind the sternomastoid muscle and across the floor of the posterior triangle of the neck. It is also vulnerable to surgical trauma during lymph node biopsy and other procedures. Lesions may result in weakness and wasting of the sternomastoid and upper part of the trapezius muscle.

XII hypoglossal nerve

The hypoglossal nerve is the motor nerve to the tongue, and its fibres originate from the hypoglossal nucleus in the medulla. The nerve fibres emerge on the ventral aspect of the medulla between olives and pyramids, and leave the skull through the hypoglossal canal to supply the muscles of the tongue (Fig. 9.27).

A unilateral lesion results in wasting of one side of the tongue. On protrusion the tip of the tongue deviates to the paralysed side. Fasciculations may be observed when the tongue lies at rest on the floor of the mouth. In bilateral lesions, the tongue may be shrunken and wasted, and protrusion may be impossible. Dysarthria and dysphagia result.

Nuclear lesions in the medulla may occur in poliomyelitis, motor neurone disease, vascular occlusions and syringobulbia. Basal meningitis, or infections or injuries of the occipital bone may affect the nerve in its infranuclear course. It may sometimes be injured by operations on the neck.

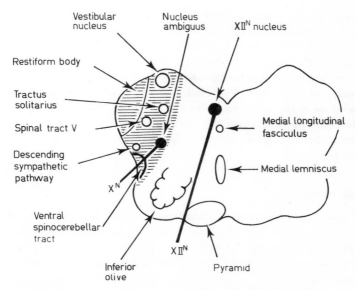

Fig. 9.27 Section of medulla, at the level of the inferior olives. Shaded area is that supplied by the posterior inferior cerebellar artery.

Bulbar palsy

Bulbar palsy is the result of weakness or paralysis of muscles supplied by the medulla, which are mainly those of pharynx, larynx and tongue, producing difficulty with speech and swallowing. Causes include acute disorders such as diphtheria, Guillain-Barré syndrome, brainstem infarction, poliomyelitis, and chronic progressive disorders such as motor neurone disease, tumours or aneurysms in the posterior fossa. Myasthenia gravis may also cause bulbar weakness.

Pseudobulbar palsy

Pseudobulbar palsy results from bilateral corticobulbar tract lesions. The palate cannot be elevated fully voluntarily, but responds briskly in the gag reflex. Speech and swallowing become slow and difficult, and the tongue appears small and cannot be protruded fully. The jaw jerk and facial reflexes are exaggerated. The patients frequently have marked emotional lability. Pseudobulbar palsy is seen particularly in hypertensive cerebrovascular disease, motor neurone disease, and multiple sclerosis, although a parasagittal tumour must always be excluded.

Brainstem disorders

The cranial nerve nuclei and their connections, the ascending and descending long tracts, and the cerebellar peduncles are all closely related to one another anatomically in the brainstem so that lesions in this area usually involve more than one structure.

The brainstem may be damaged by vascular lesions, demyelination, tumours or infections. The clinical features of brainstem disorders depend upon the anatomical site of the lesion. Common neurological manifestations of brainstem involvement are unilateral or bilateral pyramidal tract signs or sensory disturbances, associated with cranial nerve palsies.

Midbrain lesions

Lesions involving the *superior colliculi* and *tectal* region result in paralysis of vertical gaze, failure of pupils to react to light, and impairment of convergence (Parinaud's syndrome). This is most commonly seen in pineal tumours, but also occurs with multiple sclerosis and vascular lesions.

More anteriorly placed lesions of the tegmentum of the midbrain at this level may cause third nerve palsy and contralateral hemiplegia as a result of destruction of the corticospinal tracts in the cerebral peduncles (Weber's syndrome); or contralateral cerebellar ataxia and gross 'wing-beating' (rubal tremor) from involvement of the brachium conjunctivum or red nucleus, together with corticospinal tract signs (Benedikt's syndrome); or contralateral cerebellar ataxia and tremor alone (Claude's syndrome) (see Fig. 9.11).

Decerebrate rigidity results from a midbrain lesion, and is manifested by opisthotonus and extension of arms and legs. It may be caused by midbrain tumours, vascular and other lesions, or by herniation of the midbrain through the tentorial notch as a result of raised intracranial pressure.

Lesions of the pons

There may be hemiplegia and sensory disturbances on the side opposite the lesion; ataxia on the same side as the lesion as a result of damage to cerebellar peduncles; palsies in nerves VI, VII, VIII; internuclear ophthalmoplegia when the medial longitudinal fasciculus is involved; nystagmus; or Horner's syndrome. Both pupils may be small in a bilateral lesion, when consciousness is usually impaired. Spontaneous vertical eye movements ('ocular bobbing') may be observed.

The Millard-Gubler syndrome is a unilateral and/or VII nerve palsy with a crossed hemiplegia resulting from a lesion at the base of the pons.

Medulla

The lateral part of the medulla is classically affected when infarction results from lesions of the posterior inferior cerebellar artery (lateral medullary syndrome; Wallenberg's syndrome). Clinical features include: nausea, vomiting, giddiness (vestibular nucleus); hiccoughs; pain and numbness over the ipsilateral side of face (fifth nerve nucleus, descending tract of fifth nerve); dissociated sensory loss of the contralateral side of the body (spinothalamic tract); ipsilateral cerebellar ataxia (cerebellum, inferior cerebellar peduncle); dysphagia, palatal weakness, hoarseness and vocal cord paralysis (nucleus ambiguus); ipsilateral loss of taste (tractus solitarius); and ipsilateral Horner's syndrome (descending sympathetic tract).

Cerebellopontine angle tumours

Acoustic neuromas are the most common tumours in this region but meningiomas, cholesteatomas, trigeminal neuromas, and rarely aneurysms can also cause a cerebellopontine angle syndrome.

Acoustic neuromas arise from nerve VIII and unilateral nerve deafness is the chief symptom. The tumours may enlarge to involve the neighbouring nerves VII and V, causing facial paralysis and loss of sensation over the ipsilateral side of the face and a depressed corneal reflex. Ipsilateral cerebellar ataxia may result from compression of the cerebellar hemisphere, and hemiplegia and hemianaesthesia from pressure on the long tracts in the brainstem. The diagnosis should be made when the tumour is small by investigating thoroughly patients with nerve deafness.

References

Baloh R.W. and Honrubia V. (1979) *Clinical Neurophysiology of the Vestibular System*. F.A. Davis, Philadelphia.

Brodal A. (1965) *The Cranial Nerves. Anatomy and Anatomico-clinical Correlations*, 2nd edn. Blackwell Scientific Publications, Oxford.

Brodal A. (1969) *Neurological Anatomy in Relation to Clinical Medicine*, 2nd edn. Oxford University Press, Oxford.

Cogan D.G. (1956) *Neurology of the Ocular Muscles*, 2nd edn. Thomas, Springfield.

Leigh R.J. and Zee D.S. (1983) *The Neurology of Eye Movements*. F.A. Davis, Philadelphia.

10 Cerebellum

The cerebellum is situated below the tentorium cerebelli in the posterior fossa of the skull, in close relationship to the pons and medulla, and forms the roof of the fourth ventricle (Fig. 10.1). Its chief functions are to control muscle tone, posture and movement.

The cerebellum is composed of a median vermis and two lateral hemispheres, but, functionally and phylogenetically, it has been divided into: flocculonodular lobe (archicerebellum), and corpus cerebelli which is in two parts (i) anterior lobe (palaeocerebellum), (ii) posterior lobe (neocerebellum) (Fig. 10.2).

The flocculonodular lobe is connected mainly with the vestibular nuclei, the anterior lobe mainly with spinal pathways and the posterior lobe predominantly with the cerebral cortex (Figs 10.3–10.5).

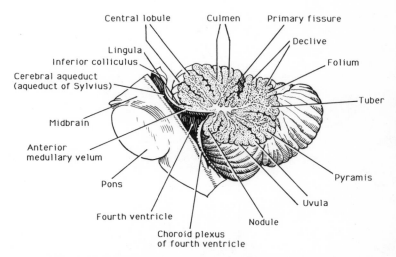

Fig. 10.1 Sagittal section of the cerebellum showing its relationship to the fourth ventricle and brainstem. (Modified from Chusid, *Correlative Neuroanatomy and Functional Neurology*, 19th edn, 1985, with permission of Lange Medical Publications.)

Fig. 10.2 Anatomical divisions of the cerebellum. (Modified from Chusid, *Correlative Neuroanatomy and Functional Neurology*, 19th edn, 1985, with permission of Lange Medical Publications.)

Fig. 10.3 Connections of the flocculonodular lobe of the cerebellum.

Fig. 10.4 Connections of the posterior lobe of the cerebellum.

Fig. 10.5 Connections of the anterior lobe of the cerebellum. DCT, dorsal spinocerebellar tract; VCT, ventral spinocerebellar tract; VN, vestibular nuclei; RF, reticular formation; RN, red nucleus.

The cerebellar cortex has a uniform structure throughout the cerebellum and is divided into three main zones: an outer molecular layer (basket cells, stellate cells, parallel fibres from granular cells, and dendrites of Purkinje cells); Purkinje cell layer; and a granular layer (granule cells, Golgi II cells).

Deep in the white matter lie the paired intracerebellar nuclei, viz. the globose and emboliform nuclei, the dentate nuclei and the fastigial nuclei.

Connections of the cerebellum

Flocculonodular lobe

The flocculonodular lobe (archicerebellum) is intimately connected with the vestibular nuclei by way of the inferior cerebellar peduncle (restiform body) (Fig. 10.3).

Posterior lobe

Descending fibres from the frontal, parietal and temporal lobes of the cerebral cortex project to the posterior lobe of the cerebellum (neocerebellum) and also to its anterior lobe by way of the pons and middle cerebellar peduncle. The efferent pathway from the Purkinje cells of the cerebellar cortex projects to the dentate nuclei, thence to the red nucleus and lateral ventral nucleus of the thalamus back to the frontal cortex. This cortico-ponto-cerebello-dentato-rubro-cortical pathway provides a feedback mechanism for the control of active movement, and also plays a part in the programming of movement (Fig. 10.4).

Anterior lobe

The anterior lobe (palaeocerebellum) receives an input from the spinal afferent system through the superior and inferior cerebellar peduncles and also via the inferior olive by way of the olivo-cerebellar tract (Fig. 10.5).

Muscle spindle afferents (Group Ia, II) and Golgi tendon organ afferents (Group Ib) project to the anterior lobe by way of the dorsal and ventral spinocerebellar tracts. Information derived from these proprioceptive sources is integrated in the cerebellar cortex, and efferent pathways from the cerebellum pass to the reticular formation, red nucleus and vestibular nuclei. The reticulospinal, rubrospinal and vestibulospinal tracts regulate posture and control movement by influencing activity in alpha and gamma motoneurones in the spinal cord segments (Fig. 10.5).

The cerebellar cortex organizes information derived from a variety of afferent sources and each cerebellar hemisphere regulates motor activity on the ipsilateral side of the body.

The only efferent output from the cerebellar cortex is by way of the Purkinje cells, which have a purely inhibitory action on the subcortical intracerebellar nuclei and vestibular nuclei. By means of patterned in-hibition, the cerebellum regulates slow movements by feedback to the motor cortex. It controls ballistic movement by programming the timing and duration of contraction in antagonistic muscle groups so that a target is reached with precision. The physiological role of the cere-bellum becomes apparent when its normal function is impaired by disease or injury.

Clinical features of cerebellar disorders in man

Muscle tone

Muscle tone is reduced on the ipsilateral side with unilateral cerebellar lesions; with more extensive lesions of the cerebellum, there is gener-alized hypotonia. The hypotonia may be demonstrated in several ways: (i) as a diminished resistance to passive movement, (ii) as a greater range of motion of the joints when the limbs are passively shaken, (iii) if the arms are held vertically and the hands allowed to fall loosely the hand may fall passively into a position of greater flexion on the affected side, (iv) if the arms are held outstretched and gently tapped there may be wider excursions of the affected limb, (v) with the patient lying supine, the heel on the affected side may be easily pressed against the buttock when the legs are flexed, (vi) if the knee jerk is tested with the leg hanging freely over the side of the bed, the leg may make several oscillations after the deep tendon reflex has been elicited — pendular knee jerks.

It seems that the hypotonia is caused by decreased muscle spindle responsiveness to stretch consequent upon a depression of fusimotor activity.

Static tremor

A slow, coarse tremor may be apparent when the arms are held out-stretched.

Disturbance of posture

There may be a tendency to fall to one side or another (to the side of the lesion if there is unilateral cerebellar involvement), or forwards or backwards when standing with the feet together. This is not materially affected by eye closure. The head may be held in a rotated position, with the occiput toward the affected side of the cerebellum.

Ataxia of gait

There is a wide based, staggering gait; with unilateral lesions, patients deviate and stagger to the affected side, and rotate to that side when walking on the spot with the eyes closed.

Disorders of movement

(a) There is delay in starting and stopping movements (which gives rise to the 'rebound phenomenon').

(b) Dysmetria. There is a disorder of the rate, regularity, range and force of compound movements.

(c) Decomposition of movements. The movements are jerky and broken up into their component parts, instead of appearing smooth and free-flowing. Dysmetria and decomposition of movements may be demonstrated clinically by finger-nose and heel-knee tests.

(d) Dysdiadochokinesis. There is an inability to carry out alternating movements with rapidity and regularity.

(e) Intention tremor. Intention tremor is an important sign because it occurs principally in disorders of the cerebellum or its connections. It is demonstrated in the upper limb by asking the patient to put his finger on his nose. There may be no tremor at rest or on commencement of the movement, but a coarse oscillating tremor develops as the finger approaches its target. Similar tests can be carried out on the lower limbs (see Chapter 2).

Speech

Speech is slurred and often broken up into syllables (scanning speech).

Nystagmus

Nystagmus is usually most marked on deviating the eyes to the side of the lesion. It is due to involvement of the vestibular connections of the cerebellum.

Localization of lesions within the cerebellum

Lateral hemisphere lesions

Lesions of the neocerebellum result in hypotonia, dysmetria, dysdiadochokinesis, past pointing, pendular knee jerks on the side of the lesion, and a tendency to stagger and to fall to the affected side. Primary tumours such as astrocytomas, metastatic tumours and abscesses are more common in the lateral hemispheres than in the midline of the cerebellum.

Anterior lobe lesions

Lesions of the anterior lobe cause ataxia of gait and of lower limbs and trunk, with relatively little involvement of upper limbs. The most common cause of this type of midline cerebellar lesion is alcoholic cerebellar degeneration, which affects the anterior superior surface of the cerebellum selectively.

Flocculonodular lobe

Lesions of the flocculonodular lobe (e.g. medulloblastoma) cause marked ataxia of gait and disturbance of balance or truncal ataxia.

Causes of cerebellar disorders

Developmental anomalies
Basilar impression — deformation of the posterior fossa by invagination of the odontoid process through the foramen magnum. Arnold–Chiari malformation — a tongue of cerebellum protruding through the foramen magnum, and downward displacement of the medulla into the cervical canal.

Cerebellar atrophies
Familial cerebellar degeneration. Olivo-ponto-cerebellar atrophy. Carcinoma — cerebellar degeneration as a remote manifestation of a distant malignancy. Alcohol.

Infections
Abscess. Viral encephalitis, especially chicken pox.

Toxins
Anticonvulsants. Alcohol.

Metabolic
Myxoedema. Hypoglycaemia. Heat-stroke.

Vascular
Occlusion of posterior inferior, anterior inferior, or anterior cerebellar arteries. Haemorrhage.

Trauma

Tumours
Intracerebellar (e.g. astrocytoma, medulloblastoma, metastases). Extracerebellar (e.g. meningioma, acoustic neuroma).

Demyelination
Multiple sclerosis.

References

Gilman S. (1986) Cerebellum and motor dysfunction. In *Diseases of the Nervous System*, pp. 401–22. Eds A.K. Asbury, G.M. McKhann and W.I. McDonald. W.B. Saunders, Philadelphia.

Gilman S., Bloedel J.R. and Lechtenberg R. (1981) *Disorders of the Cerebellum*. F.A. Davis, Philadelphia.

11 Extrapyramidal Disorders

The extrapyramidal system

By definition, the extrapyramidal system consists of all descending motor pathways that do not run through the pyramids of the medulla. Extrapyramidal fibres arise from almost all areas of the neocortex, particularly the sensorimotor area, and project from the cortex to subcortical nuclei, the basal ganglia, and then to the brainstem and spinal cord. Extrapyramidal activity is finally expressed through reticulospinal and vestibulospinal pathways in the medulla which are influenced by the basal ganglia and cerebral cortex (Fig. 11.1).

The extrapyramidal system complements the function of the pyramidal tract in controlling *tone*, *posture* and *movement*. It is responsible for maintenance of the upright posture and for movements involving axial (neck and trunk) and proximal muscles, while the pyramidal tract promotes abduction of the upper limbs, flexion of the lower limbs and movement of distal muscles. When normal subjects stand upright with upper limbs flexed and lower limbs extended to resist the force of gravity they are in a posture of reflex standing determined primarily by vestibulospinal and associated pathways. When this posture is assumed voluntarily, it can be interrupted by pyramidal activity so that the limbs are then placed in a position appropriate for a planned movement, which requires active extension of the upper limbs and flexion of the lower limbs (as in walking). When the posture of reflex standing is assumed involuntarily as the result of damage to the cortex or basal ganglia it cannot be altered voluntarily and is then called the 'decorticate posture' or 'dystonia-in-extension' (extension here referring to the lower limbs). This posture may be seen as the end result of damage to the caudate nucleus and putamen as in Huntington's chorea and dystonia musculorum deformans. When this posture involves one side only as a result of contralateral cerebral damage it is known as the *hemiplegic posture*. In Parkinson's disease, on the other hand, selective damage to the nigrostriatal system may lead finally to a posture in which both upper and lower limbs are flexed ('dystonia-in-flexion').

Fig. 11.1 Extrapyramidal system. Fibres of cortical origin project to basal ganglia (BG), reticular formation (RF), vestibular nuclei (VN) and other subcortical structures. Extrapyramidal projections to the lower motor neurone are mainly through the reticulospinal and vestibulospinal tracts.

When one pyramidal tract is destroyed in primates (including man), the extrapyramidal system remaining intact, movements may recover 85% of their power and dexterity, leaving slight weakness of upper limb abductors and lower limb flexors, and loss of discrete movements of the digits.

The basal ganglia

The basal ganglia include the *caudate nucleus* and *putamen* (neostriatum) which receive afferents from the cerebral cortex, midline thalamic nuclei and reticular formation, and project to the *globus pallidus* (palaeostriatum) and *substantia nigra*. Output from the neostriatum passes through the globus pallidus to make the following connections:
(a) To the ventrolateral (VL) nucleus of the thalamus (Fig. 11.2) (i) directly by the ansa lenticularis and fasciculus lenticularis which loop across the internal capsule; (ii) indirectly via part of the substantia nigra

Fig. 11.2 Cortico-strio-thalamo-cortical loop. Corticofugal fibres concerned with the programming and feedback of movement pass to the caudate nucleus (CN) and putamen (P). The caudate nucleus and putamen project to the ventrolateral nucleus of the thalamus (Th) via the globus pallidus (GP) and substantia nigra (SN), and thence to the motor cortex (MC).

(zona reticulata) which is homologous to the pallidum and, like the pallidum, projects to the VL nucleus.

(b) To the medial nuclei of the thalamus, which are a rostral extension of the reticular formation (Fig. 11.3).

(c) To the subthalamic nucleus (Fig. 11.4).

Since the VL nucleus of the thalamus projects back to the sensorimotor cortex, connection (a) forms a circuit (cortex → striatum → thalamus → cortex) which can play a part in the programming of movement or in feedback control of movement in progress. The connections with the reticular formation on the other hand form a loop concerned with the control of muscle tone through the reticulospinal and vestibulospinal pathways.

There are two other regulatory circuits of clinical significance (Fig. 11.4): (a) Part of the substantia nigra (zona compacta) gives origin to the nigrostriatal pathway which regulates activity in the caudate and putamen through a dopaminergic pathway. Degeneration of this pathway is one of the main causes of symptoms in Parkinson's disease. There is a reciprocal pathway from the striatum to substantia nigra using

Fig. 11.3 Reciprocal connection with the reticular formation. Fibres from the caudate nucleus (CN) and putamen (P) project through the globus pallidus (GP) to medial thalamic nuclei and thence to the reticular formation (RF) of the midbrain. Fibres from substantia nigra (SN) also feed into the same pathway. The reticular formation projects back through medial thalamic nuclei to the caudate nucleus. This circuit appears to be concerned with the control of muscle tone.

GABA as a transmitter. (b) The *subthalamic nucleus* projects to globus pallidus by an inhibitory pathway which presumably regulates the control of axial and proximal movements by the striatum, because damage to this pathway releases flinging and rotary movements (ballistic movements) of the limbs which are seen unilaterally in the clinical condition of *hemiballismus*.

Extrapyramidal syndromes

Parkinson's disease

In 1884, Professor Charcot wrote to a Dr Nunn, saying 'I have seen your patient suffering from paralysis agitans, Parkinson's disease as I call it'. This is the first time that the name of James Parkinson was applied to

Fig. 11.4 Reciprocal connections modulating basal ganglia function. (i) With the subthalamic nucleus (ST). Interruption of this pathway causes hemiballismus. (ii) With the substantia nigra (SN). Striatonigral neurones inhibit SN cells by the release of GABA. The nigrostriatal pathway, which uses dopamine as a transmitter and degenerates in Parkinson's disease, inhibits cells in the putamen (P) and caudate nucleus (CN). GP, globus pallidus; Th, thalamus.

'shaking palsy' although his monograph was published 67 years before, in 1817. Parkinson's description of the disease reads 'involuntary tremulous motion, with lessened muscular power, in parts not in action and even when supported with a propensity to bend the trunk forwards, and to pass from a walking to a running pace: the senses and intellects being uninjured'. The description remains valid except the last phase, since recent studies have demonstrated intellectual failure in some patients.

Aetiology

This condition is a degenerative disorder of the central nervous system affecting primarily the substantia nigra. The most common form of Parkinson's disease (affecting about 1/1000 of the population) is *idiopathic* (*paralysis agitans*); it usually appears after the age of 50 and a family history may be obtained in 4–16% of cases. The *postencephalitic* form which followed a worldwide epidemic of encephalitis lethargica after World War I is now very rare. Parkinson's disease may also be *secondary* to drugs (especially dopamine antagonists such as phenothiazines, alpha methyl dopa and reserpine), carbon monoxide, methyl bromide, manganese poisoning and MPTP, a contaminant of synthetic heroin. A similar extrapyramidal syndrome may follow head injury and vertebrosilar ischaemia.

Pathophysiology

The most constant pathophysiological feature of idiopathic Parkinson's disease is the loss of melanin-containing cells in the substantia nigra and locus coeruleus as well as the dorsal motor nucleus of the vagus nerve. Degenerative changes may also be found in the cortex and corticostriatal fibres. Ehringer and Hornykiewicz reported in 1960 that the concentration of dopamine in the neostriatum was reduced in Parkinsonian patients. There is a relative hyperactivity of striatal cholinergic mechanisms.

The failure of dopaminergic control of basal ganglia mechanisms permits rhythmic synchronous bursts of impulses to traverse the pathway from cortex to basal ganglia to thalamus to cortex, which then propagate down the pyramidal tract as a tremor rhythm and may be transmuted into an alternating tremor by the reciprocal innervation of spinal cord mechanisms. Alternating tremor can thus be controlled by stereotactic lesions in the globus pallidus or ventrolateral nucleus of the thalamus which interrupt this circuit. The same lesions reduce rigidity in 70% of cases because of the reciprocal connections with the reticular formation which promote hyperactivity of alpha and gamma motor neurones in Parkinson's disease.

Clinical features

The onset is insidious with symptoms and signs comprising slowness in initiating and performing movement (bradykinesia), tremors, cog-wheel rigidity, loss of righting reflexes, and autonomic disturbances.

Bradykinesia   Failure to swing one or both arms on walking. Difficulty in moving the feet, leading to a shuffling gait. 'Freezing' (shuffling of the feet on one spot) on attempting to walk. Writing becoming slower and smaller (micrographia). Loss of expression from face and voice.

Tremors Exaggeration of physiological tremor at 8–9 Hz. Postural tremor at 6 Hz. Action tremor at either of the above frequencies. Resting (alternating) tremor at 4–5 Hz.

An understanding of the different varieties of tremor is of practical importance because an action tremor may be present in Parkinson's disease for many years before the classical alternating ('pill-rolling') tremor appears, and its detection, particularly if it is unilateral, helps to confirm the diagnosis of Parkinson's disease. The frequency of the beats of cog-wheel rigidity is determined by the type of tremor dominating anterior horn cells at the time of examination.

Cog-wheel rigidity The increased resistance to stretch on passive movement at a joint in Parkinson's disease is uniform throughout the range of movement and has a plastic or 'lead-pipe' quality. It shows little of the dynamic (velocity-sensitive) quality that characterizes the spasticity of upper motor neurone lesions. Flexor spasms and the clasp-knife phenomenon are never observed in Parkinson's disease since they depend on the release of the reflex effects of flexor reflex afferent fibres which, in contrast to spasticity, remain under brainstem control in Parkinson's disease. The rigidity is interrupted by a tremor mechanism (commonly that of action tremor) to impart a ratchet or cog-wheel sensation, to the examiner as the limb is moved.

Glabella tap sign may be present (failure to inhibit eye-blinking when the forehead is tapped repeatedly).

Tendon jerks are usually within the normal range and plantar responses remain flexor.

Posture Body posture becomes progressively more flexed as the condition advances.

Loss of righting reflexes Patients tend to fall and are unable to make normal corrective movements to retain balance. They may tend to totter forwards with increasing speed (*festination of gait*) or fall backwards (*retropulsion*).

Autonomic disturbances Postural hypotension; excessive salivation; and urgency of micturition in 25% of patients.

Change in intellect and mood Depression is common in Parkinson's disease and dementia may occur later in the disease as a result of the associated cerebral atrophy.

Treatment

Principles It is important to keep the patient as active as possible and avoid unnecessary bed-rest, to treat the mental depression which is commonly associated, and to start any form of drug therapy in low dosage because of the risk of mental confusion in the elderly.

The aim of medical treatment is to dampen cholinergic activity, which is relatively excessive in Parkinson's disease, and to increase dopaminergic activity which is diminished. The latter is accomplished by giving levodopa, the precursor of dopamine, since dopamine does not cross the blood–brain barrier. Levodopa is now commonly administered with a decarboxylase inhibitor to prevent the transformation of levodopa to dopamine in the gastrointestinal tract or elsewhere in the body and thus to permit higher blood levels of levodopa and greater entry through the blood–brain barrier. There is some controversy as to whether levodopa therapy is best started early in the disorder or deferred until essential to preserve freedom of movement. There is general agreement that treatment should be maintained at the lowest possible dosage to prevent if possible the development of the 'on-off' phenomenon (oscillation between bradykinesia and dyskinetic side-effects of levodopa therapy). It is advisable for the initiation and maintenance of treatment to be supervised by a neurologist. Treatment may be started with an anticholinergic drug, or with amantadine which releases dopamine from body stores. Levodopa or the dopamine agonist bromocriptine may then be added later in the course of the disorder if required.

Pharmaceutical agents used in the management of Parkinson's disease
(a) Anticholinergic (atropine-like) drugs.   An example is benzhexol (Artane), available in 2 mg and 5 mg tablets. Dosage is best started at 1 mg three times daily which, if it is well tolerated, can be increased slowly up to 5 mg three times daily. Side-effects include mental confusion, dry mouth, blurred vision and difficulty in starting micturition. Anticholinergic drugs are usually contra-indicated in glaucoma.
(b) Dopaminergic agents.   *Amantadine* (Symmetrel). 100 mg capsules, usually given as one in the morning and one at midday as it may cause excitability and insomnia if given later in the day.

Levodopa. This may be given on its own (Laradopa) as 500 mg capsules, increasing the dose slowly to a total of 4 g daily if necessary. It may cause gastrointestinal irritation and some months are required before the full effect becomes apparent.

More commonly, levodopa is now given in combination with a decarboxylase inhibitor (see Chapter 23). Dosage is usually increased slowly from 50–100 mg three times daily to a maximum of 1 g daily which may be divided into 4–8 doses if necessary to avoid fluctuation in blood levels.

Side-effects include postural hypotension and involuntary movements usually of mouth, tongue and extremities (dyskinesia).

Bromocriptine. Bromocriptine is a dopamine agonist with a long half-life which may be given in low dosage (2.5 mg to 40 mg daily) alone or in conjunction with a levodopa preparation. It has also been used in larger doses of 40–60 mg daily. Its long half-life permits daily dosage and helps reduce the 'on-off' phenomenon.

Deprenyl. This inhibitor of monoamine oxidase B reduces the breakdown of dopamine and is a useful addition to levodopa therapy in resistant cases.

Choreoathetosis

Two major types of movement disorder, chorea and athetosis are distinguished but frequently they occur together and are described as choreoathetosis.

Chorea consists of involuntary, continuous, rapid, irregular, jerky movements which affect face, tongue, lips, trunk and limbs, chiefly in their distal parts. Voluntary actions may be severely interrupted and impaired by choreiform movements. The precise site of the lesions causing chorea is not certain, although there is evidence that the caudate nucleus is involved.

Athetosis is an instability or fluctuation of posture which commonly affects the hands, arms and face, and less commonly the lower limbs. The movements are slow and writhing ('mobile spasm') and an alternation between two basic postures is usually recognizable; namely pronated forearm, flexed wrist, flexed metacarpophalangeal joints and extended fingers, and supinated forearm, extended wrist and abducted fingers. The characteristic posture of the foot is inversion and plantar flexion. Athetosis is often associated with lesions of the putamen.

Causes of choreoathetosis

Both types of involuntary movement are often seen together even in conditions labelled as chorea. Choreoathetotic movements are a feature of the following disorders.

Sydenham's (rheumatic) chorea This is an immune disorder most commonly affecting young women, which follows weeks after a streptococcal sore throat in a manner similar to rheumatic fever. Since the course is benign, autopsy studies are few but cellular infiltration has been reported in cortex, basal ganglia and cerebellum. It usually resolves spontaneously over a period varying from 1 week to several years. Pure choreiform movements are often seen in this condition.

Huntington's chorea   Huntington's disease is an hereditary progressive dementia, preceded by or associated with choreoathetotic movements, which is inherited as an autosomal dominant characteristic. The age of onset is usually between 30 and 50 years. The caudate nucleus atrophies and neuronal degeneration can also be demonstrated in frontal cortex and putamen. Gamma-aminobutyric acid (GABA), glutamic acid decarboxylase (GAD), and the synthesizing enzyme for acetylcholine, choline acetyltransferase (CAT) are depleted in Huntington's disease. There is no evidence that dopaminergic neurones are released from inhibitory influence but nevertheless there seems to be undue sensitivity of neurones to dopamine. Involuntary movements are made worse by levodopa and are reduced by dopamine-blocking agents such as phenothiazines and butyrophenones (e.g. haloperidol) or by catecholamine-depleting agents such as reserpine or tetrabenazine. Medication does not alter the progressive dementia. The gene has been localized to chromosome 4, and the risk of acquisition can be determined with about 96% accuracy.

Senile chorea   A similar clinical picture to Huntington's disease may be observed in some ageing patients without a family history. The relationship, if any, to Huntington's disease is obscure.

Cerebral palsy   Infants subjected to hypoxia or other causes of diffuse brain damage *in utero*, at birth, or in early childhood may have choreoathetosis, upper motor neurone signs and intellectual impairment in varying combinations. The main pathological changes are periventricular lesions in the white matter, although signs of old cortical infarction may also be seen. Since mental ability may be normal, every attempt should be made to assess these children accurately so that they can be given every educational opportunity.

Rh incompatibility with resulting haemolytic jaundice can cause damage to the basal ganglia (*kernicterus*) because unconjugated bilirubin passes through the blood–brain barrier. The clinical picture resembles cerebral palsy with the addition in some cases of bilateral nerve deafness.

Encephalitis in early childhood may also produce a similar syndrome.

Metabolic disorder Wilson's disease (hepatolenticular degeneration) is a rare deficiency of the copper-binding protein coeruloplasmin in the plasma, with an autosomal recessive inheritance. Copper is deposited in the putamen, thalamus and basal nuclei of the cerebellum, in the liver and in the outer margin of the cornea where it can be seen as a brown band at the corneo-scleral junction (Kayser-Fleischer ring), and is excreted in excess in the urine. The neurological signs produced include choreoathetotic movements, cerebellar disturbance, a coarse postural tremor of the abducted arms ('wing-beating' or 'red nucleus' tremor) and development of dystonia-in-extension. The patients also have progressive cirrhosis of the liver and often aminoaciduria. Progress of the disease may be slowed by using penicillamine or chelating agents to help rid the body of excess copper.

Choreoathetosis may also be seen as a sequel to hypoxia or as a symptom of uraemic, hepatic or hypercapnic encephalopathy.

Drug-induced dyskinesias Some phenothiazines such as fluphenazine (Stelazine), triethylperazine (Torecan), prochlorperazine (Stemetil) and metoclopramide (Maxolon), and some butyrophenones, such as haloperidol (Serenace), can cause acute dystonic reactions shortly after they are injected or taken orally. The reactions may consist of akathisia (motor restlessness), the assumption of a dystonic posture, or choreoathetotic movements. The reaction is rapidly reversed by the injection of an anticholinergic agent such as benztropine methane sulphonate (Cogentin), 2 mg intravenously.

The prolonged use of such drugs may cause the gradual development of a choreoathetotic syndrome (*tardive dyskinesia* — 'tardive' because it is slow in developing) which responds poorly to withdrawal of the offending drug and to drug treatment.

Dystonia

Dystonia is a disorder in which attempted voluntary movement leads to tonic contraction of antagonistic muscle groups causing part or whole of the body to assume an abnormal posture. At first such postures are transient but may become permanent as 'dystonia-in-flexion' or 'dystonia-in-extension'. Dystonic features may become superimposed on other basal ganglia disorders and may progress until the patient remains in a permanent dystonic posture.

The idiopathic dystonias may be considered as general (dystonia musculorum deformans) or focal.

Dystonia musculorum deformans

Dystonia musculorum deformans (torsion spasm) is a rare disorder which may be familial (autosomal dominant or recessive) or sporadic. This disorder starts in childhood with 'freezing' of gait similar to that seen in Parkinson's disease or with twisting movements of the head and trunk. Speech becomes slow and the mouth may be held open by excessive muscular contraction. The limbs become rigid so that writing and other hand movements are impaired and the patient has to swing the pelvis to place the lower limbs for walking. A form which fluctuates in severity during the day has been reported to respond to levodopa, but generally treatment with dopamine-blocking agents gives greater, although modest, benefit. Anticholinergic drugs, phenothiazines and butyrophenones are also used. Stereotactic thalamotomy is helpful in some cases.

Focal dystonias

These are much more common than dystonia musculorum deformans and are frequently mistaken for manifestations of hysteria, particularly as the symptoms of all basal ganglia disorders become worse with emotional stress. No neuropathological changes have been described at autopsy and the focal dystonias are considered to be disorders of neurotransmitters localized to various parts of the basal ganglia. They are made worse by levodopa (indeed they may appear as side-effects when levodopa is given to patients with Parkinson's disease) and benefit to some extent from dopamine-blocking agents. Some patients improve with biofeedback training and psychological management.

Recognized focal dystonias include (i) *Writer's cramp*. Writing is distorted by contraction of antagonistic muscles in the hand and forearm. Undue muscle contraction extends proximally to the shoulder girdles. Various occupational cramps, which affect muscle groups used in skilled movements, such as the playing of musical instruments, are similar in nature to writer's cramp. (ii) *Torticollis*. The head and neck turn involuntarily to one side. The condition is at first spasmodic but may become permanent. *Retrocollis* (extension of the neck) and *anterocollis* (flexion of the neck) are related disorders. (iii) *Blepharospasm* and *orofacial dyskinesia*. Involuntary closure of the eyelids (blepharospasm) and grimacing movements of the mouth and face (orofacial dyskinesia) may occur as separate entities or in association, in which case the combination is known as *Miege's syndrome*. The onset is usually in late middle age or in the elderly. Blepharospasm has been reported to respond to clonazepam therapy but this has not been our experience. Phenothiazines such as thioridazine (Melleril) are helpful in some cases. Injection of dilute botulinum toxin into the periocular muscles relieves the condition for some months and may be repeated as necessary. Similar injections into neck muscles are useful in the management of torticollis. (iv) *Laryngeal dystonia.* Spasm of the larynx on attempting to speak gives a forced grating quality to the voice resembling that of chronic laryngitis.

Gilles de la Tourette syndrome

Multiple tics, resembling the common habit spasms of anxiety, may develop in children or adolescents to the point where loud explosive grunting or coughing noises interrupt normal conversation or relaxation. Later an expletive may be uttered during the compulsive expiration, which has led to the condition being considered a psychiatric manifestation in the past. It should probably be classified as a variation of focal dystonia. It usually responds at least partially to therapy with clonidine, clonazepam, haloperidol or pimozide (Orap).

Hemiballismus

Destruction of the subthalamic nucleus or its connections by infarction or haemorrhage causes the sudden onset of wild involuntary movements involving the proximal muscles of the limbs on the opposite side of the body. The disorder usually subsides with time but can be controlled with dopamine-blocking agents and abolished by stereotactic thalamotomy on the side contralateral to the ballistic movements.

Paroxysmal choreoathetosis

This is an unusual and intriguing syndrome in which the assumption of a dystonic posture or involuntary choreoathetotic movements appear transiently and intermittently. There are two forms. (i) *Paroxysmal kinesigenic choreoathetosis.* Attacks are induced by startle or movement, hence the term 'kinesigenic', and last for 1–3 min at a time. The condition may be familial or sporadic. (ii) *Paroxysmal dystonic choreoathetosis.* A rare familial condition, in which the attacks persist much longer, for hours rather than minutes, and are precipitated by excitement or the taking of alcohol or coffee. The cause is unknown but appears to be a periodic disinhibition of basal ganglia mechanisms.

The kinesigenic form responds to anticonvulsants such as carbamazepine (Tegretol) and phenytoin (Dilantin). The dystonic form does not improve with these agents but does appear to be prevented by clonazepam (Rivotril).

Tremor

Not all tremors are caused by diseases of the basal ganglia but the problem is logically reviewed at the conclusion of a chapter on these disorders. Tremors commonly encountered are classified below.

Physiological tremor

Maintenance of posture or voluntary movement is accompanied by a tremor of about 10 Hz (7–12 Hz) in normal people. This is characterized by synchronous contraction of antagonistic muscles and is accentuated by anxiety, fatigue, thyrotoxicosis and circulating noradrenaline. It is also increased early in Parkinson's disease, in which case an action tremor at about 6 Hz is usually evident as well.

Senile tremor

As age advances, the frequency of physiological tremor slows to 6–7 Hz and may become more conspicuous, particularly during a slow movement such as drinking a glass of water.

Familial or 'essential' tremor

This may take different forms but commonly resembles an exaggerated physiological tremor or senile tremor with some accentuation on attempting fine coordinated movements. It is improved temporarily by taking alcohol, or more consistently by taking regular medication with the beta-blocking agent propranolol (Inderal), the barbiturate anticonvulsant primidone (Mysoline), or by taking drugs of the benzodiazepine series such as diazepam (Valium).

Parkinson's disease

In the early stages of Parkinson's disease, synchronous tremors of 6–9 Hz may be evident but later in the disorder, contractions alternate between antagonistic muscles at 4–5 Hz, giving rise to the characteristic resting tremor. The thumb may also move rhythmically over the pulp of the index finger, a movement known as 'pill-rolling' tremor.

Midbrain tremor ('red nucleus' or 'wing-beating' tremor)

This is a coarse alternating movement seen in the outstretched or abducted upper limb with lesions of the midbrain or of the dentatorubral pathway from cerebellum to midbrain. It may be seen in metabolic disorders such as Wilson's disease, or more commonly, in multiple sclerosis or vascular disease.

Intention tremor

Damage to the cerebellar hemispheres or their dentatorubral projections gives rise to a tremor at 3–8 Hz which increases in amplitude as the limb approaches its target in coordinated movement. Intention tremor (and the midbrain tremor which occasionally accompanies it) can be diminished by medication with clonazepam and abolished by stereotactic thalamotomy.

Asterixis

This is the so-called 'flapping tremor' of the outstretched hands seen in hepatic encephalopathy and other metabolic disorders. It is not strictly a tremor but is the result of episodic inhibition of muscles sustaining posture against gravity.

Hysteria

Coarse tremors may be observed in hysterical cases, sometimes with jactitations of the limbs resembling an epileptic fit to the unseasoned eye, and sometimes with a calculated and precise misplacement of the finger on approaching a target which could suggest intention tremor to an unwary observer.

References

DeLong M.R. and Alexander G.E. (1986) Organization of basal ganglia. In *Diseases of the Nervous System*, pp. 379–93. Eds A.K. Asbury, G.M. McKhann and W.I. McDonald. W.B. Saunders, Philadelphia.

Findley L.J., Gresty M.A. and Halmagyi G.M. (1981) Tremor, the cogwheel phenomenon and clonus in Parkinson's Disease. *J. Neurol. Neurosurg. Psychiat.* **44**, 534–46.

Hornykiewicz O. (1976) Neurohumoral Interactions and Basal Ganglia Function and Dysfunction. In *The Basal Ganglia*, pp. 269–80. Ed. M.D. Yahr. Raven Press.

Lance J.W. and McLeod J.G. (1981) *A Physiological Approach to Clinical Neurology*, 3rd edn. Butterworths, London.

Martin J.B. and Gusella J.F. (1986) Huntington's disease. Pathogenesis and management. *New Engl. J. Med.* **315**, 1267–76.

12 Focal Cerebral Lesions and Tumours

Lesions in different anatomical sites of the cerebral hemispheres have specific clinical features.

Frontal lobes

The frontal lobes are usually divided into the precentral region or motor cortex, and the prefrontal region (Fig. 3.9).

Prefrontal lobes (areas 9, 10, 11, 12, 13)

Information concerning the function of the prefrontal lobes comes largely from studies on patients with gunshot wounds and other injuries, and from patients subjected to prefrontal leucotomies. Clinical features of prefrontal changes are:

(a) Personality change — loss of insight; carelessness about appearance, dress and habits; shallowness of emotion; jocularity, facetiousness and making simple jokes and puns; lowering of intelligence, difficulty in concentrating, impairment of judgement and of grasping situations as a whole; difficulty in changing from one mental activity to another, repetition of phrases (*palilalia*) or words (*echolalia*).

(b) Grasp reflex — this is a primitive reflex, normally found only in infants, that consists of flexion of thumb and fingers on stroking the skin of the palm between thumb and index fingers. It becomes disinhibited in frontal lobe lesions.

(c) Sucking and pouting reflexes — these are other primitive reflexes that become disinhibited. Lightly stroking the lips produces a sucking movement, and tapping the closed lips causes contraction of the circumoral muscles ('pouting').

(d) Tonic innervation or tonic perseveration is a persistence of muscular contraction such as may be seen in a failure to relax the grip or repetition of an action after it has become inappropriate.

(e) Incontinence of urine and faeces.

(f) Epileptic seizures may be a symptom of frontal lobe tumours, infarcts and other lesions.

(g) Unilateral anosmia may result from meningiomas of the olfactory groove (see p. 113).

(h) Unilateral optic atrophy with papilloedema in the other eye (Foster-Kennedy syndrome) may result from frontal lobe tumours (see p. 119).

(i) Incoordination and ataxia may occur (Brun's frontal ataxia), probably caused by interruption of the cortico-ponto-cerebellar pathways (Chapter 10).

(j) Frontal apraxia of gait may result from bilateral parasagittal frontal lesions. The patient can make walking movements while lying down but is unable to walk spontaneously while standing.

Precentral region (areas 4 and 6)

Lesions in the precentral region of the frontal lobe involving the motor areas characteristically cause:

(a) Weakness in the form of a hemiparesis or monoparesis, depending on the site of the lesion.

(b) Dysphasia if the posterior part of the third frontal gyrus in the dominant lobe is involved (Broca's aphasia) (Fig. 12.1).

(c) Jacksonian fits with an irritative lesion. If the frontal adversive fields (area 8) are involved, the head and eyes will deviate usually to the opposite side.

Temporal lobes

Temporal lobe lesions cause the following.

Visual field defects

Disease of either temporal lobe may result in a superior quadrantanopia on the opposite side due to involvement of Meyer's loop (Chapter 9; Fig. 9.4).

Aphasia

Disease involving the posterior part of the superior gyrus of the dominant temporal lobe will result in a Wernicke's or central aphasia, i.e. difficulty in understanding spoken or written words, and jargon aphasia (Fig. 12.1).

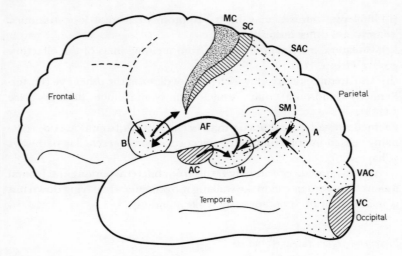

Fig. 12.1 The neurological basis for language skills.

Speech. The basic speech circuit comprises: primary auditory cortex (AC), association cortex (Wernicke's area, W), arcuate fasciculus (AF), Broca's area (B), motor cortex (MC) and corticobulbar pathways. This circuit is responsible for repetition of the spoken word and is influenced by input from dominant frontal and parietal lobes.

Language: The supramarginal (SM) and angular (A) gyri form a language integrating centre with afferent inflow from the visual cortex (VC) and visual association cortex (VAC) for the interpretation of the written word, from Wernicke's area for the spoken word and from the sensory cortex (SC) and sensory association cortex (SAC) for kinaesthetic information. Connections between the language integrating centre and the motor cortex are also responsible for writing and other motor skills.

Epilepsy

The patient may suffer from complex partial seizures (pp. 230–1).

Hearing defects

Hearing is bilaterally represented in the transverse convolutions of Heschl in the superior gyrus (Fig. 12.1). Hearing defects are very rare and are encountered only with bilateral temporal lobe lesions.

Memory disturbances

The hippocampal region of the temporal lobes is essential in the memory process for the acquisition of new information. Bilateral hippocampal lesions result in severe memory defects, characterized by an inability to consolidate information. Unilateral lesions do not cause disturbance of memory.

Emotion

Emotional disturbance, such as sudden outbursts of anger, may be features of temporal lobe lesions.

Parietal lobes

Lesions of the parietal lobes cause the following.

Disorders of tactile sensation

Since the parietal lobes are the main receiving area in the cerebral cortex for the somatic sensory pathways, lesions involving this area (3, 1, 2)of the brain may result in sensory impairment. Irritative lesions may result in 'sensory fits' of a Jacksonian type. Destructive lesions result in impairment of spatial and discriminative aspects of sensation — 'cortical sensory loss' — in which there may be impairment of two-point discrimination, astereognosis (inability to recognize shape and texture of an object), impairment of position sense and tactile inattention or extinction (failure to recognize a stimulus on one side of the body when both sides are touched simultaneously). Other modalities of sensation may be intact.

Disorders of motility

Hypotonia and wasting of the contralateral limbs may occur rarely — 'parietal lobe wasting'.

Visual defects

Homonymous hemianopia or visual inattention to the opposite half-fields may be detected. Opticokinetic nystagmus is impaired to the side of the lesion (p. 132).

Gerstmann's syndrome

In dominant parietal lobe lesions there may be agraphia (impairment of ability to write), acalculia (inability to calculate), finger agnosia (inability to recognize and identify fingers correctly), and left-right disorientation. These four clinical features are together known as Gerstmann's syndrome. There may also be dyslexia (difficulty in reading) and an ideomotor apraxia.

Apraxias

Apraxia is the inability to carry out a purposive movement, the nature of which the patient understands, when there is no accompanying motor impairment, sensory loss, or ataxia. The following types of apraxia are recognized.

Ideomotor apraxia   The patient has no difficulty in formulating the idea of a simple act that he is instructed to carry out, but he finds himself unable to execute it. Thus he may not protrude his tongue to command, but will spontaneously lick his lips; he cannot make a fist, but he can grasp an object spontaneously.

Ideational apraxia   This is a disturbance of more complicated tasks, e.g. lighting a cigarette, pouring out a glass of water.
   Ideomotor and ideational apraxia are caused by lesions of the parietal or frontal lobes, particularly in the dominant hemisphere.

Dressing apraxia   This is a difficulty in putting on garments correctly and is usually due to a lesion of non-dominant parietal lobe.

Constructional apraxia   This is a disorder of visuo-spatial function. The patient has difficulty in drawing common objects (e.g. a bicycle), or making designs from matchsticks or blocks. This is caused most commonly by a non-dominant parietal lobe lesion, but may also be seen in dominant lobe lesions.

Disorders of the body image

These are usually associated with lesions of the non-dominant parietal lobe. There may be a unilateral neglect — motor, sensory or visual — of the opposite side. Hemiplegic patients may ignore the paralysed limb (*autotopagnosia*) or even deny their hemiplegia (*anosognosia*). The non-dominant parietal lobe appears to serve the same function for visuo-spatial integration as the dominant parietal area does for speech.

Occipital lobes

Lesions of the occipital lobes characteristically result in visual field defects (Figs 9.5, 9.6). A destructive lesion involving the whole of one occipital lobe will result in a congruous contralateral homonymous hemianopia. Bilateral occipital lesions will result in cortical blindness with preservation of pupillary reflexes, a clinical state that may be difficult to distinguish from hysteria. Some patients may be unaware of, or deny, their blindness (*Anton's syndrome*). Lesions involving visual association areas 18 and 19 will result in inability to recognize faces or objects even though they can be seen (visual agnosia). Irritative lesions of the primary visual cortex may cause epileptic fits with an unformed visual aura — coloured or flashing lights — while formed hallucinations may be evoked from the visual association cortex.

Speech disorders

Anatomy and physiology

In 1861 Paul Broca pointed out that disturbed language output results from damage to a specific area of the brain — the posterior part of the third frontal gyrus of the dominant hemisphere (*Broca's area*). This area lies immediately in front of the muscles of the face, jaw, tongue, palate and larynx, i.e. the muscles of speech production.

In 1874 Carl Wernicke described an area at a site in the left hemisphere in the posterior aspect of the superior temporal gyrus adjacent to the auditory area. Damage to Wernicke's area results in loss of comprehension of speech.

Wernicke's and Broca's areas are interconnected by a bundle of nerve fibres — the arcuate fasciculus. When a word is heard, the output from the primary auditory area is received by Wernicke's area. If the word is spoken, the pattern is transmitted from Wernicke's area to Broca's area and then on to the motor area that controls the speech muscles. Interconnections with other areas in the parietal lobe of the dominant hemisphere are necessary for reading and spelling (Fig. 12.1).

The left hemisphere is dominant (i.e. concerned with language function) in over 90% of right-handed people. In left-handed people the left hemisphere is dominant in more than 50%, so that only a small number of people have a dominant right hemisphere.

Motor pathways for speech

The descending motor pathways for articulation are (i) the corticobulbar tracts which arise from the precentral gyrus and travel to the V, VII, XII nerve nuclei and to the nucleus ambiguus, and (ii) the corticospinal tracts to the diaphragm and intercostal muscles. The cerebellum and basal ganglia also exert a controlling influence over articulation.

Development of speech

The understanding of language begins in infancy well before speech emerges. The successful development of speech requires normal hearing.

Vocalization develops during the first year. The first words normally appear at about 12 months of age. By 2 years of age the average child will understand several hundred words and regularly use some 200. However very wide individual variations occur and a few normal children may use only a dozen or so words by their second birthday.

The average age of first using two-word phrases is 18 months and by 2 years of age nearly 90% are using simple word sequences. Girls are usually slightly more advanced than boys in language development.

Delayed speech

There may be a delay in learning to speak up to the age of 3–3½ years (developmental delay)that is not explicable by anatomical, auditory, intellectual, metabolic or psychiatric disturbance. This condition is compatible with a high order of intelligence, and motor and social development proceeds normally. Comprehension of speech is frequently normal. A positive family history is often obtained. Boys are affected about three times as frequently as girls, and a proportion of them have difficulty later in learning to read, write and spell. A speech therapist should be consulted for children who are not putting two words together by 2 years of age. However, mental retardation is the commonest cause of delayed speech; defective hearing, brain damage and psychiatric disturbances are other important causes.

Developmental dyslexia

Developmental dyslexia is a difficulty in learning to read, displayed by normally intelligent children who have intact sensory mechanisms and are not emotionally disturbed, and has been estimated to affect 10–20% of primary school children. There is no underlying structural lesion of the brain. In addition to the reading disability the child often has difficulty in writing.

Aphasia

Aphasia is a disorder of the higher language functions of speech. Several different types are recognized.

Expressive (Broca's) aphasia

Lesions of Broca's area in the posterior part of the third frontal gyrus of the dominant hemisphere produce a *non-fluent aphasia*. There is a sparse output of words and the speech that is produced is uttered slowly, with great effort and poor articulation. It lacks small grammatical words and endings, so that it takes on a telegraphic quality. Asked about the weather, such a patient may say 'sunny', and if urged to produce a full sentence he may say 'weather . . . sunny'. Broca's aphasia is usually associated with hemiparesis. The speech lacks normal rhythm and melody (*dysprosody*).

Receptive (Wernicke's) aphasia

Wernicke's aphasia is caused by lesions in Wernicke's area in the posterior part of the superior temporal gyrus in the dominant hemisphere. It is a *fluent aphasia*: the patient produces well articulated, long phrases or sentences with a normal grammatical skeleton, having normal rhythm and melody. Speech may be faster than normal. However, the speech is abnormal in that its content is defective. Circumlocution, nonspecific words (e.g. 'thing'), and incorrect words are all used. The term *paraphasia* is used to describe the substitution of syllables, or words which are often nonsense words. Patients with Wernicke's aphasia have a failure of understanding and an inability to repeat simple phrases. Comprehension of written language, as well as spoken language, may be affected.

Nominal aphasia

This is an inability to name objects. It occurs in the recovery phase of most aphasias, but also in a pure form with lesions in the parieto-temporal region of the dominant hemisphere.

Transcortical aphasia

The ability to repeat test phrases is intact because the basic speech circuit of Wernicke's area-arcuate fasciculus-Broca's area is spared. There is impairment of spontaneous speech because the input from frontal and parietal areas of the cortex to the basic speech circuit is prevented by a transcortical lesion. This disturbance is most often encountered with a 'watershed infarction' at the junction of middle cerebral and anterior cerebral arterial territories.

Conduction aphasia

This is a result of a lesion localized to the arcuate fasciculus. Spontaneous speech is impaired by substitutions, but comprehension is good in contrast to transcortical aphasia. Repetition is impaired.

Dysarthria

Dysarthria is a disorder of articulation. The motor pathways for the production of sound are disordered but the patient has no difficulty in comprehending or expressing himself in writing or by gesture. He has no difficulty in the mental formation of words or sentences, nor any difficulty in the handling of verbal symbols.

Dysarthria must be distinguished from aphasia. A simple rule of thumb is that when speech is transcribed, correct English sentences are produced in dysarthria but not in dysphasia.

Upper motor neurone lesions

Since muscles of articulation are bilaterally innervated, it is usually necessary to damage both corticobulbar tracts in order to cause spastic dysarthria. Bilateral capsular lesions, brainstem vascular lesions, motor neurone disease and multiple sclerosis are some of the possible aetiological factors in this type of speech disorder.

On examination, the jaw jerk and facial reflexes are found to be brisk; the tongue may appear small and contracted and cannot be fully protruded; swallowing may be affected, and there may be emotional lability.

The complete syndrome is sometimes called *pseudobulbar palsy*. The speech is slow and forced, the patient has particular difficulty in enunciating labial and dental sounds.

Extrapyramidal lesions

In Parkinson's disease, articulation is slow and slurred and the speech is monotonous and lacking inflection.

In both spastic dysarthria and extrapyramidal disorders, but especially the former, there is usually poor coordination of the respiratory muscles and diaphragm, so that speech is often in short breathless sentences.

In athetosis (for example, cerebral palsy from birth hypoxia) the voice is slow, consonants are pronounced poorly if at all and speech is accompanied by inappropriate involuntary movements.

Cerebellar lesions — ataxic dysarthria

Coordination of articulation becomes impaired. The speech is slow and slurred and there may be an unnatural separation of syllables ('scanning speech'). This is seen in multiple sclerosis, Friedreich's ataxia and cerebellar degenerations.

Lower motor neurone lesions

The tongue becomes wasted, the palate weak, and the facial muscles incapable of adequate movements. This condition is known as *bulbar palsy*, and can occur in poliomyelitis, motor neurone disease, medullary tumours and syringobulbia. Phonation may also be impaired, and the speech becomes slurred and indistinct. Labial sounds usually suffer first. In palatal palsy, speech has a nasal quality and there is difficulty with sounds such as 'ing' and 'egg'.

Myopathies

Myopathies and myasthenia result in similar disturbances to bulbar palsy.

Dysphonia

This is an inability to approximate the vocal cords normally for speech or coughing, giving a husky or gravelly quality to the voice. It occurs in bulbar palsy, recurrent laryngeal nerve paralysis and rarely as a focal dystonia which may be mistaken for an hysterical manifestation.

Examination of the patient with a speech disorder

Disorders of speech are distressing to the patient since they severely impair the ability to communicate and to play a useful role in life. It requires patience on the part of the physician to make contact with such patients and to elucidate the nature of their condition.

The first thing is to determine the nature of the speech disorder. If it is aphasia, the following outline of examination is useful.

(a) Ensure that the patient is alert, mentally clear and intellectually unimpaired. Examination periods should be limited to 15–20 minutes because fatigue interferes with responses to tests.

(b) Determine whether the patient is right- or left-handed when writing, playing games or sighting guns.

(c) Estimate the probable level of education for reading and writing.

(d) Note spontaneous speech. Is it slow or fast, fluent or non-fluent? Is it grammatical?

(e) Can the patient understand spoken language? Test the response to simple verbal commands, e.g. put out your tongue, close your eyes, put your right hand on your head, touch your right ear with your left hand.

(f) Can he repeat words and sentences?

(g) Can he read? Make sure he has no organic visual defects. Test his understanding of simple written commands. Give him sentences from newspapers and books to read.

(h) Can he write? Test his spontaneous writing, e.g. name and address, letter to a relative. See if he can write to dictation and copy.

(i) Can he name common objects?

Cerebral tumours

Cerebral tumours may present as focal cerebral lesions, or with signs of generalized disturbance of cerebral function.

The cranial cavity is a closed, inexpansible box and tumours produce symptoms because they grow and expand inside this space, and compress and displace the brain and other structures.

There are many different types of tumours — benign and malignant — and the prognosis for recovery in many of these is very good if they are treated early, so that it is important to recognize the symptoms and diagnose and treat the underlying tumour. Next to stroke, tumour is the most common type of intracranial disease.

Frequency of different types of tumours

The frequency of different types of tumours depends on the age group studied and the method of selection. Approximate frequencies of tumours for all ages are: glioma 45%; meningioma 15%; metastases 15%; pituitary tumours and craniopharyngioma 10%; acoustic neuroma 7%; others 8%.

Some tumours are more frequent in the young (e.g. medullo-blastoma, pinealoma), and some are more frequent in older age groups (e.g. glioma, meningioma, metastases).

The symptoms of cerebral tumours

These depend upon the site in the brain, the type of tumour and its rate of expansion. The chief clinical features are:

Change in mental function

Dullness, apathy, lack of initiative, abnormal social behaviour, forget-fulness, personality change, weakness, tiredness, dizziness are common symptoms. These features are seen especially in frontal and temporal lobe, and corpus callosum tumours.

Headaches

These are usually dull, non-pulsatile, worse in the morning and aggrav-ated by sneezing, coughing or head movement. They are caused by dis-placement of blood vessels and other pain-sensitive structures or by raised intracranial pressure. About 30% of patients with cerebral tumour experience headaches as a presenting symptom.

Vomiting

This is usually associated with a headache and may be projectile in type, without associated nausea.

Epilepsy

About 20–50% of patients with cerebral tumour are subject to seizures which may be either focal or generalized in type.

Raised intracranial pressure

The symptoms of raised intracranial pressure are headache, vomiting, mental changes, unsteadiness of gait and incontinence. Papilloedema may be seen on examination of the optic fundi.

Raised intracranial pressure may give rise to *false localizing signs* which are unrelated to the anatomical site of the tumour. These include sixth nerve palsy, uncal herniation with third nerve palsy (pp. 194–5), ataxia and pyramidal tract signs.

Focal signs

Tumours, regardless of type, may give rise to focal signs appropriate to their anatomical site in the cerebral hemispheres, i.e. frontal, temporal, parietal or occipital.

Specific signs

Some tumours have specific signs, for example:

Acoustic neuroma   These arise from the auditory nerve in the cerebello-pontine angle. They cause deafness and in more advanced cases lower motor neurone facial weakness, sensory loss on the face, absent corneal reflex, and incoordination on the side of the lesion.

Pituitary tumours   These may be non-secreting (e.g. chromophobe adenoma) or hormone-secreting causing acromegaly, Cushing's disease, or hyperprolactinaemia. They often extend superiorly from the posterior fossa, compressing the optic chiasm and causing bitemporal hemianopia (Figs 9.2, 9.3, 9.6). Sometimes they invade the cavernous sinus laterally involving the third, fourth, fifth (first and second division) and sixth nerves (Fig. 9.12).

Sphenoidal wing meningiomas   If they are near the superior orbital fissure they cause unilateral exophthalmos and involve nerves III, IV and V (first division). A more medially placed tumour may compress the optic nerve as it passes through the optic foramen causing unilateral loss of vision and optic atrophy.

Olfactory groove meningioma   These rise from the floor of the anterior cranial fossa and compress the olfactory bulb causing anosmia. As they expand they may cause a frontal lobe syndrome.

Pinealoma   These arise from the pineal gland and compress the tectal region of the midbrain causing Parinaud's syndrome (p. 130) (dilated pupils which do not react to light; impairment of upward gaze and vergence), and raised intracranial pressure.

References

Adams R.D. and Victor M. (1985) *Principles of Neurology*, 3rd edn. McGraw-Hill, New York.

Benson D.F. (1979) *Aphasia, Ataxia and Agraphia*. Churchill-Livingstone, New York.

Critchley M. (1953) *The Parietal Lobes*. Hafner, New York and London.

Geschwind N. (1965) Disconnection syndromes in animals and man. *Brain* **88**, 237–94; 585–644.

Geschwind N. (1970) The organization of language and the brain. *Science* **170**, 940–4.

Kartesz A. (1979) *Aphasia and Associated Disorders. Taxonomy, localisation and recovery*. Grune and Stratton, New York.

13 Coma and Other Disturbances of Consciousness

Consciousness

There is no entirely satisfactory definition of consciousness but clinically it means the state of awareness of self and environment. Coma is a state in which a patient is unaware of self and environment, and does not respond to external stimuli.

The structures which are most important in maintaining the state of consciousness are the cerebral cortex and the reticular formation. The reticular formation (from the Latin reticulum, meaning 'a net') consists of large and small cells with their connections which are scattered throughout the brainstem from the medulla to the thalamus. It is divided anatomically into the brainstem and thalamic reticular formation. All the major sensory pathways project to the reticular formation which is influenced by, and in turn can modify, the sensory input to the brain. One of the most important functions of the reticular formation is in arousal and in maintaining wakefulness. The part of the reticular formation most concerned with this function is the ascending reticular formation (reticular activating system) in the midbrain and thalamus which projects diffusely to the cerebral cortex. Destruction of the ascending reticular activating system causes coma and stimulation of it will cause wakefulness in an experimental animal (Fig. 13.1).

Definition of altered states of consciousness

Various grades of impaired or clouded consciousness are recognized and are loosely defined as follows.

Alert wakefulness

The subject is fully orientated in time and place, and responds immediately and appropriately to stimuli.

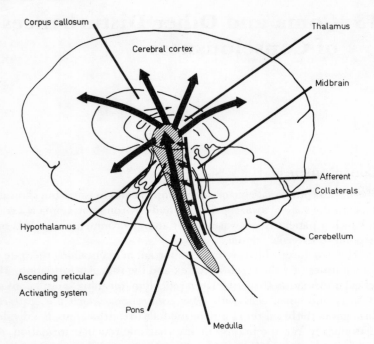

Fig. 13.1 Ascending reticular activating system. (Modified from Lindsay, 1958, *Reticular Formation of the Brain*, Little Brown, New York.)

Confusional states

The patient has difficulty in concentrating and thinking. There is lack of attentiveness, some degree of disorientation in time and place, distractibility, and impairment of memory.

Delirium is a confusional state in which the patient is anxious, excited, agitated and often hallucinating. *Delirium tremens* is a condition seen in heavy drinkers who suddenly cease drinking alcohol, often because of admission to hospital. It is characterized by agitation, mental confusion, hallucinations, tremor, sweating and tachycardia. It may be fatal if not recognized and treated. Other neurological complications of alcoholism include withdrawal seizures (p. 233), peripheral neuropathy (pp. 68–9), cerebellar degeneration (p. 161), Wernicke's encephalopathy (pp. 198, 208), and Korsakoff's psychosis (p. 208).

Confusional states and delirium are common and may be caused by a variety of aetiological factors which include drugs, fevers, infections, metabolic disorders, cerebral anoxia, head injuries, cerebrovascular disease and post-epileptic states.

Lethargy

The subject is drowsy and indifferent to his surroundings but responds to verbal stimuli. 'Obtundation' is a term also used to describe such a state of dull indifference.

Stupor

The patient is unconscious but can be aroused by pain and can give some sort of voluntary response.

Coma

The patient is unrousable and primitive reflexes only are present.

These are all terms to describe different states of unconsciousness, but in examining a patient it is most important to make a detailed record of the patient's clinical state and reactions rather than to use one of these labels, which are capable of different interpretations by different observers. The Glasgow coma scale is widely used in the assessment of level of consciousness; scores are assigned for (i) eye opening, (ii) verbal response, and (iii) motor response.

There are certain conditions that should be recognized clinically in which there is a state of chronic alteration in consciousness.

Akinetic mutism   is a condition in which the patient is immobile, and has the external appearance of being alert but does not speak, move spontaneously or respond to external stimuli. It may result from bilateral frontal lobe lesions, diffuse cerebral damage following cardiac arrest, asphyxia, carbon monoxide poisoning and lesions around the third ventricle. The reticular-cortical pathways are interrupted but the corticospinal pathways are often spared. *Chronic vegetative state* is a term used to describe a similar condition following severe head injury. A condition that may be confused with coma and which it is important to recognize is the *locked-in syndrome*; consciousness is preserved but the limbs and lower cranial nerves are paralysed, and the patient is mute. The patient can usually indicate his understanding and awareness by blinking and by vertical eye movements. The lesion is most commonly an infarct of the ventral aspect of the base of the pons; it interrupts the motor pathways but spares the tegmentum, including the reticular formation and the supranuclear pathways for eye-movement control.

Mechanisms of coma

Coma is caused by either or both: (i) widespread lesions affecting the whole of the cerebral cortex, e.g. metabolic processes, head injury; (ii) lesions involving directly or indirectly the ascending reticular formation in the thalamus, midbrain or pons.

Small focal cerebral and medullary lesions are not sufficient in themselves to cause coma; it is necessary for the reticular formation to be involved before consciousness is impaired.

Anatomically, the site of lesions causing coma can be subdivided as follows: supratentorial (15%); infratentorial (15%); diffuse disorders affecting the brain (70%), e.g. drug intoxication, metabolic disturbances.

Placing the disorder into one of these three categories can usually be effected by careful clinical examination.

Supratentorial lesions

Supratentorial lesions causing coma are those which involve the reticular formation directly or indirectly, such as cerebral haemorrhages, tumours, abscesses, large infarcts, subdural haematomas and head injury.

The reticular formation may be involved by bilateral deep structural lesions in the region of the thalamus, or by unilateral hemisphere lesions that have resulted in displacement of the brain, impairing secondarily the deep-lying structures. The cerebral hemispheres are confined in a rigid compartment bound by the skull and tentorium cerebelli. When a mass lesion expands, the brain tissue shifts across the midline or downwards in the following ways (Fig. 13.2).

Cingulate herniation   The cingulate gyrus is displaced medially under the falx, causing compression of blood vessels; cerebral ischaemia, venous congestion and oedema result.

Central or transtentorial herniation   The brainstem is forced downwards through the tentorial notch, compressing the diencephalon and midbrain, and interfering with the blood supply to the brainstem.

Uncal herniation   The uncus and hippocampal gyrus of the medial temporal lobe are forced through the tentorial notch, compressing the midbrain and stretching the third nerve on the same side. The *uncal syndrome* consists of a third nerve palsy and signs of midbrain compression. It is most commonly seen after head injuries and intracranial

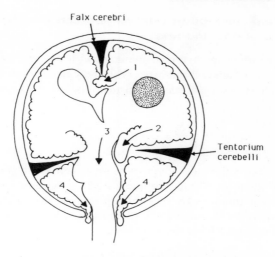

Fig. 13.2 Effect of supratentorial expanding lesions on cerebral structures. The cingulate gyrus may be herniated beneath the falx cerebri (cingulate herniation) (1), a portion of temporal lobe may be compressed between brainstem and margin of tentorial notch (2), or the brainstem may be displaced downwards through the tentorial opening (central herniation) (3). In expanding infratentorial lesions, or after injudicious lumbar puncture in the presence of raised intracranial pressure, the cerebellar tonsils may herniate through the foramen magnum (4). (From Lance and McLeod, 1981, with permission of Butterworths, London; modified from Plum and Posner, 1980.)

haemorrhage which is rapidly expanding. The presence of a unilateral dilating pupil in a patient after a head injury should prompt immediate neurosurgical intervention.

Subtentorial lesions

The posterior fossa is a tight inelastic compartment, so that expanding lesions such as tumours or abscesses may cause pressure on brainstem structures with upward herniation of the brain through the tentorial notch and downward herniation of the cerebellar tonsils giving rise to medullary compression and death. Lumbar puncture is highly dangerous and should be avoided when there is raised intracranial pressure from any cause and in the presence of space occupying lesions, particularly those in the subtentorial region, because it may precipitate herniation through the foramen magnum.

Metabolic and other diffuse cerebral disorders causing disturbances of consciousness

Metabolic disturbances, hypoxia, meningitis, drugs and toxins may affect the whole of the cerebral cortex or the reticular formation or both structures. There are usually no focal neurological signs on examination.

Drugs

Drug overdosage is the most frequent cause of coma in a general hospital. The drugs most commonly implicated are barbiturates, benzodiazepines, phenothiazines, tricyclic antidepressants, alcohol and opiates (pin-point pupils are characteristic). Chemical screening tests on blood and urine will usually identify the poison.

Disorders of carbohydrate metabolism

(a) *Diabetic coma* may be due to diabetic ketoacidosis; the patients are dehydrated and have deep sighing respirations (Kussmaul breathing). Hyperosmolality usually accompanies diabetic ketoacidosis but hyperosmolar coma, in which dehydration is a prominent feature, may occur without the presence of ketoacidosis. It should be noted that there are many causes of elevated blood sugar in coma other than diabetes mellitus, e.g. cerebral infarction, head injury, meningitis.

(b) *Lactic acidosis.* This usually occurs in patients receiving metphormin or other oral hypoglycaemic agents. The patients have Kussmaul breathing but no ketosis. Blood glucose may or may not be elevated.

(c) *Hypoglycaemia* is often accompanied by signs of sympathetic overactivity — sweating, tachycardia, dilated pupils and tremor. If untreated it will cause irreversible brain damage since brain cells require both glucose and oxygen for their metabolism. The brain contains a reserve of only about 10 g of glucose and when this supply is depleted it metabolizes its own tissues. Hypoglycaemic coma most commonly results from overdose of insulin, sulphonylureas or phenformin in diabetics but can also be caused in non-diabetics by alcohol, fasting, pancreatic islet cell tumours, hypothyroidism and hypopituitarism.

Hypoxia

The brain consumes about 15–50% of the total body oxygen requirements. Brain cells are permanently damaged after 4 min of anoxia; the hippocampus and cerebellum are particularly susceptible. The most common causes of cerebral hypoxia are cardiorespiratory arrest, chronic obstructive airways disease, pneumonia and prolonged hypotension.

Uraemia

Encephalopathy in chronic renal failure is due to multiple causes which include metabolic acidosis, electrolyte disturbances and dehydration. The acidosis is aggravated by hypotension, infection, fluid depletion and sodium restriction.

Calcium disorders

Hypocalcaemia may occur in association with uraemia or in hypoparathyroidism; tetany and fits are common. Hypercalcaemia may be seen in primary hyperparathyroidism, cancer and prolonged immobilization; dehydration, weakness, anorexia, nausea and vomiting are common features.

Hepatic coma

Patients with hepatic encephalopathy usually first develop delirium or mental confusion and then gradually lapse into coma. A characteristic feature is *asterixis*, a periodic inhibition of muscles causing lapses in posture of the hands at the wrists when the arms are outstretched and the hands dorsiflexed with fingers extended (hepatic flap). The most important factors responsible for the development of hepatic coma are the effects of ammonia and other nitrogenous products or toxic substances such as short chain fatty acids, indoles and drugs normally detoxified in the liver. Hypoglycaemia may also contribute.

Hypothyroidism

Primary or secondary hypothyroidism may cause coma associated with hypothermia. Coma may be precipitated by cold, infection or withdrawal of thyroid drugs. Clinical features include the generalized facial characteristic of myxoedema, low body temperature and delayed relaxation of the ankle jerks. *Hypothermia* in the absence of hypothyroidism can produce almost identical clinical signs.

Water intoxication

Water intoxication may be caused by excess water ingestion, abnormal hypotonicity (e.g. Addison's disease), decreased water excretion (e.g. nephrotic syndrome), inappropriate antidiuretic hormone (ADH) secretion due to central cerebral lesions, or occur as a paraendocrine phenomenon associated with carcinoma. Inappropriate ADH secretion is quite common as a cause of confusion in patients with cerebral lesions and may also develop in patients treated with carbamazepine (Tegretol). The resulting hyponatraemia should be treated cautiously.

Thiamine deficiency

Wernicke's encephalopathy is caused by a thiamine deficiency and is most commonly seen in alcoholics. It may be precipitated by increased glucose intake in malnourished alcoholics who have recently been admitted to hospital. The clinical features are mental confusion, nystagmus, bilateral sixth nerve palsies, and ataxia; about 80% of patients also have a peripheral neuropathy. Pathological changes are found in the mamillary bodies, the thalamus and hypothalamus, around the third ventricle, around the aqueduct in the midbrain, and the floor of the fourth ventricle. Treatment is 100 mg of thiamine intravenously daily for several days and then regular oral vitamin supplements. It should be noted that patients with Wernicke's encephalopathy may present in coma as well as with mental confusion.

Infection

Meningitis and encephalitis may cause coma and other disturbances of consciousness. Neck stiffness is a characteristic sign of meningitis in the early stages of the illness but may be absent in a deeply comatose patient.

Epilepsy

Complex partial seizures cause mental confusion and disturbances of consciousness. Postictal state, and status epilepticus should be considered in the differential diagnosis of coma.

Subarachnoid haemorrhage

Subarachnoid haemorrhage may cause loss of consciousness with or without focal neurological signs. Neck stiffness is usually present, although it may be absent in a deeply comatose patient.

Evaluation of the comatose patient

The questions that must be answered when examining a comatose patient are:
(a) Where is the lesion? Is the disease focal due to a structural lesion, or is it diffuse, due to a metabolic or toxic process? If it is focal, is it supratentorial or infratentorial?
(b) Is the condition progressing, improving or remaining static?
(c) What is the specific pathological process?

While history taking, physical examination and investigations are proceeding to answer these questions, it is essential first to protect the brain by maintaining adequate oxygenation, blood pressure, circulation and metabolism with intravenous glucose and fluids.

History

If possible, obtain from observers a description of the onset of the coma, when the patient was last seen, his behaviour at the time, and his habits. Is he diabetic or epileptic? Is he alcoholic or an abuser of drugs? Has he had psychiatric treatment or emotional disturbances? Has he been treated for renal, cardiac, thyroid or respiratory disease?

Physical examination

All details should be carefully recorded.

General

Pay attention to breath, colour, skin, pulse, blood pressure, scalp wounds, temperature, urine, and examination of heart, lungs and abdomen. A slowing pulse and rising blood pressure may indicate increasing intracranial pressure. A stiff neck indicates meningeal irritation due to meningitis or subarachnoid haemorrhage.

Neurological

State of consciousness　Pay particular attention to, and record carefully the details of, the patient's level of consciousness. Can he be aroused? Does he respond to pain? Is he confused, agitated or delirious? Assess his level of consciousness using the Glasgow coma scale (p. 193). These details will be important in gauging progress.

Respiration　Record the rate and rhythm of respiration. Different types of respiration are recognized in comatose patients.

(a) Cheyne-Stokes. This is a periodic waxing and waning of the amplitude of respiration and usually implies either a metabolic disturbance or bilateral deep hemisphere lesions, e.g. in the thalamus or internal capsule, but sometimes as low as the level of the pons.

(b) Central neurogenic hyperventilation. Automatic overbreathing which indicates a lesion of the reticular formation in the low midbrain or pons, or a metabolic disturbance such as diabetic ketosis or salicylate poisoning.

(c) Apneustic respiration. There are prolonged pauses in the respiratory cycle at full inspiration. The condition is seen in pontine lesions, usually infarction.

(d) Ataxic respiration. There is a completely irregular respiratory pattern; the condition, which is seen in medullary lesions, has a very poor prognosis.

The pupils   Note the size, shape, equality and reaction to light of the pupils. Specific abnormalities to observe are the fixed dilated pupil of a third nerve palsy; Horner's syndrome which may be seen in hypothalamic and brainstem lesions; the pupils fixed in mid-position and unreactive to light in midbrain lesions; the pin-point pupils of pontine lesions or narcotic overdosage.

Ocular movements   Remember that in unconscious patients with supratentorial hemisphere lesions the eyes are deviated towards the side of the lesion, whereas in pontine lesions the eyes are deviated away from the side of the lesion. It follows that if the patient is hemiplegic the eyes are deviated away from the hemiplegic side in supratentorial lesions, and towards the hemiplegic side in pontine lesions.

In an unconscious patient eye movements can and always should be tested reflexly in order to assist in the localization of the level of the lesion. There are two main reflexes:

(a) The oculocephalic reflex which is elicited by brisk head movements (doll's eye phenomenon). Rotation of the head to one side causes the eyes to turn to the opposite side. Flexion of the neck makes the eyes roll upwards and extension of the neck causes the eyes to look downwards.

(b) The oculovestibular reflex, which is elicited by caloric irrigation. Ice cold water syringed into one ear causes the eyes to deviate to the side of the irrigation; it is a more potent stimulus of eye movements than head movement.

The oculovestibular and oculocephalic reflexes in general are present in supratentorial lesions or in metabolic causes of coma. The reflex eye movements are impaired when brainstem structures are involved.

Lateral pontine lesions result in impaired conjugate eye movements towards the side of the lesion. When the medial longitudinal fasciculus is involved in the pons or midbrain, an internuclear ophthalmoplegia will be evident. When the third nerve or its nucleus is involved, the features of a third nerve palsy will be evident on reflex stimulation. Damage to the pretectal region of the midbrain will give rise to impaired upward gaze (see Chapter 9).

Motor function   Posture of the limbs, spontaneous movements, responsiveness to painful stimuli and reflexes should be observed as these may indicate the presence and site of a focal cerebral lesion. Does the patient spontaneously or reflexly move the limbs more on one side of the body than the other? Decerebrate rigidity (extension of the neck, extension, adduction and pronation of the arms, and extension of the legs with plantar flexion of the feet) is a sign that the midbrain is involved either primarily or secondarily.

It is important to pay particular attention in comatose patients to *changes* in the patient's condition and in the observations, e.g. slowing pulse, rising blood pressure, dilating pupils.

Clinical features of metabolic disorders and other diffuse conditions causing coma

Since metabolic disorders and diffuse disease of the brain are the most common causes of coma in a general hospital it is important to recognize the clinical manifestations. In general there are no focal neurological signs.

Levels of consciousness

Changes in alertness, orientation and concentration, impairment of memory, and changes in affect and perception are common early signs of metabolic disturbances.

Respiration

Cheyne-Stokes respiration is common in metabolic disorders. Hyperventilation may result from metabolic acidosis (uraemia, diabetes, lactic acidosis or salicylates), and hypoventilation may result from metabolic alkalosis.

Pupils

The pupils usually remain responsive to light in metabolic disorders unless the patient is hypoxic or specific drugs have affected their reactions, such as atropine (causing dilated pupils), morphine, physostigmine, timolol (causing a constricted pupil) or glutethemide (pupils in mid-position).

Ocular movements

Doll's head manoeuvre and caloric stimulation produce conjugate movements of the eyes, unless the patient is in deep coma.

Motor activity

Focal neurological signs are not present except in some metabolic disturbances, particularly hypoglycaemia, uraemia and hepatic coma. Tremor, asterixis and myoclonus are common in metabolic disturbances.

Psychiatric causes of coma

It is important to remember that apparent coma may be due to hysteria or malingering. In these conditions, the respirations are usually normal in rate and depth, and the pupils react normally unless mydriatic drugs have been administered. The patient usually resists any attempt to open the eyes. Tone and deep tendon reflexes are normal, and plantar responses are flexor. Abdominal reflexes are present. Slow, roving eye movements do not occur and on caloric irrigation of the ears with ice cold water, there is no tonic deviation of the eyes to the ipsilateral side, but rather the quick-phase nystagmus to the contralateral side that is characteristic of a conscious patient.

Management of coma

The immediate management of the comatose patient is to maintain basic life support by:
(a) Clearing the airway of foreign material.
(b) Tilting the head backwards and supporting the jaw.
(c) Applying mouth-to-mouth resuscitation if necessary.
(d) Nursing in the lateral position to allow adequate drainage of saliva and vomitus.

After these emergency measures have been undertaken the patient may require advanced life support with:

(a) Oxygen therapy.
(b) Monitoring and maintenance of blood pressure.
(c) Intravenous fluids and restoration of acid–base balance.
(d) Intravenous glucose and thiamine.
(e) Careful nursing care with attention to skin, bowels, and bladder.
(f) Artificial respiration.

Investigations in coma

Neurological

CT scan or arteriography is essential if a mass lesion is suspected. Lumbar puncture is indicated only if infection or subarachnoid haemorrhage is suspected and if a space-occupying lesion has already been excluded. Note that unilateral or bilateral subdural haematomas may not be detected by CT scan and cerebral angiography may then be required to make the diagnosis.

General

Full blood count, blood glucose, serum electrolytes (note patterns of abnormality in diabetic hyperosmolar states, inappropriate ADH secretion, lactic acidosis), liver function tests, drug screen, urine examination, chest X-ray. After blood has been taken it is worthwhile injecting glucose intravenously as a routine if there is any possibility of hypoglycaemia. Similarly, 100 mg thiamine should be given parenterally if Wernicke's encephalopathy or nutritional deficiency is suspected.

Brain death

Brain death is the state in which brain tissue is damaged to such an extent that vital cerebral functions are irreversibly damaged, regardless of whether or not the heart is beating. It is now widely accepted legally as a criterion of death.

In order to make the diagnosis of brain death the patient must be deeply comatose and there should be no possibility of the coma being due to drugs, hypothermia, or reversible metabolic and endocrine causes. The diagnosis of the cause of brain death must be fully established.

The diagnostic tests for confirmation of brain death are those which establish that all brainstem reflexes are absent, namely:

(a) The pupils are fixed in diameter and do not respond to light.

(b) Corneal reflexes are absent.

(c) There are no eye movements in response to caloric irrigation of the ears (absent vestibulo-ocular reflexes).

(d) There are no reflex responses to noxious stimulation of the face.

(e) Gag reflexes are absent and there is no response to tugging an intratracheal tube.

(f) There is no spontaneous respiration when the patient is disconnected from a ventilator for a time sufficient to ensure that the carbon dioxide tension has risen above the threshold for stimulation of respiration.

(g) Brainstem reflexes remain absent despite repeated testing at intervals of up to 24 h.

Reference

Plum F. and Posner J.B. (1980) *The Diagnosis of Stupor and Coma*, 3rd edn. F.A. Davis, Philadelphia.

14 Dementia

Dementia is a progressive loss of intellectual function and memory caused by organic disease of the brain. It may be the result of primary degenerative brain disease (e.g. Alzheimer's disease, Huntington's disease) or secondary to other, potentially treatable, conditions (e.g. cerebral tumour, subdural haematoma, hydrocephalus, vascular disease and infection; see Table 14.1). It is important to distinguish intellectual failure, resulting from a single cerebral lesion, from multiple focal lesions and from a global impairment of all cortical function. Severe depressive or other psychotic states may mimic dementia.

Clinical features

Dementia may present in many ways but early features include changes in personality, apathy, faulty judgement, forgetfulness, difficulty in concentrating, irritability, disorientation, and slowness in speech and movement. These symptoms and signs, which are initially subtle, gradually become more obvious; memory becomes grossly impaired, there is loss of interest in other people and the surroundings, and there is deterioration of personal cleanliness and hygiene. In the early stages the only abnormality on neurological examination may be impairment of memory and poor performance on neuropsychological tests of intellectual function. In the later stages there is a shuffling gait, akinesia and appearance of primitive reflexes such as the grasp, snout, and sucking reflexes (Chapter 12). The presence of focal neurological signs should always alert the clinician to the likelihood of space-occupying or other focal lesions that may be treatable.

Causes of dementia

Alzheimer's disease

The association of dementia with old age has been recognized for centuries. The most common form of dementia, and the usual cause of

Table 14.1   Causes of dementia

Alzheimer's disease

Cerebrovascular disease
    Multi-infarct dementia
    Lacunar infarcts

Head injuries

Intracranial space-occupying lesions
    Tumours
    Abscesses
    Subdural haematomas

'Normal pressure hydrocephalus'

Nutritional
    Wernicke–Korsakoff syndrome
    Vitamin B_{12} deficiency
    Folate deficiency
    Pellagra

Metabolic
    Myxoedema
    Cushing's syndrome, Addison's disease
    Hypocalcaemia
    Renal, hepatic failure
    Inappropriate ADH secretion
    Intoxications

Infections
    Creutzfeldt–Jakob disease
    AIDS-dementia complex
    Neurosyphilis (general paralysis of the insane — GPI)
    Chronic meningitis, e.g. cryptococcal, tuberculous
    Abscess

Degenerative diseases
    Huntington's disease
    Pick's disease
    Parkinson's disease
    Parkinson's-dementia complex
    Spinocerebellar degenerations
    Progressive supranuclear palsy

---

senile dementia, is Alzheimer's disease originally described by Alois Alzheimer in 1907. Alzheimer's disease accounts for about 60% of cases of dementia. Prevalence is about 1% of the population aged 65 but rises steeply to about 20% of the population over the age of 80. About 50% of the nursing home population has Alzheimer's disease. As well as age, genetic factors play a part in the aetiology since there is a familial incidence of the disease. It may be significant that adults with Down's syndrome have similar neuropathological changes to those with Alzheimer's disease.

The characteristic pathological features consist of:
(a) Cortical atrophy and loss of cells, particularly the large neurones.
(b) Neurofibrillary tangles in cortical neurones, consisting of paired helical filaments that are argyrophilic (taking up silver stains).
(c) Neuritic or senile plaques are degenerating nerve terminals with a central core of amyloid. A major protein component of the amyloid (A4) is coded on chromosome 21. The number of neuritic plaques correlates with the severity of the dementia.

Depletion of chemical transmitters, particularly acetylcholine, may play an important part in the mental changes of Alzheimer's disease. There is a reduction in cholinergic activity in the brain and a loss of neurones in the major cholinergic projections to the cerebral cortex from the basal nucleus of Meynert in the substantia innominata. Some other neurotransmitters are also depleted but not to the same extent nor as consistently as the cholinergic markers. Treatment of patients with cholinergic drugs, such as oral tetrahydroaminoacridine, has had some success in temporarily improving the intellectual function and memory.

Pick's disease

This is a rare condition that is indistinguishable clinically from Alzheimer's disease. It is characterized pathologically by atrophy, mainly of the frontal and temporal lobes, and the presence of abnormal silver-staining material (Pick bodies) in swollen cortical cells.

Huntington's disease (see p. 172)

Multi-infarct dementia

Repeated cerebral infarcts will produce dementia. The degree of dementia is related to the amount of tissue destroyed. Usually there is a history of stepwise deterioration of intellectual function.

Wernicke-Korsakoff syndrome

Wernicke's encephalopathy (p. 198) is frequently associated with Korsakoff's psychosis. They are both most commonly caused by thiamine deficiency in chronic alcoholics, and are together known as the Wernicke-Korsakoff syndrome. Korsakoff's psychosis is characterized by severe impairment of memory and an inability to acquire new information. Frequently the memory defects are disguised by confabulation, i.e. fanciful invention or fabrication of information to take the place of that which has been forgotten. There is also accumulating evidence that alcoholics may develop cognitive impairment due to frontal lobe degeneration in addition to the Wernicke-Korsakoff syndrome.

AIDS-dementia complex (p. 267)

Management

A careful history from the patient, relatives and friends is essential. A progressive dementia must be distinguished from acute confusional states due to metabolic and other diffuse cerebral disorders (p. 196–8). Careful enquiry should be made about a history suggestive of stroke (multi-infarct dementia), head injuries, headaches and fits (space occupying lesions), and drug or alcohol abuse. Careful testing of the mental state should be performed and supplemented by more detailed neuropsychological tests. Physical examination should be directed towards a search for focal lesions and evidence of systemic disease. Laboratory investigations should include CT scan, chest X-ray, EEG, full blood count and ESR, serum folate and Vitamin B_{12} levels, thyroid and liver function tests, serum calcium, blood sugar, HIV antibodies, screening test for syphilis, and CSF examination.

Treatment will depend on the underlying cause, the most common cause being Alzheimer's disease for which there is no specific therapy. Supportive treatment of patient and relatives plays a major part in management.

References

Katzman R. (1986) Alzheimer's disease. *New Engl. J. Med.* **314**, 964–73.

Wells C.E. (1977) *Dementia. Contemporary Neurology Series.* Philadelphia, F.A. Davis.

Wilcock G.K. (1988) Alzheimer's disease — Current issues. *Quart. J. Med.* **66**, 117–24.

15 Cerebral Vascular Disease

The term 'cerebral vascular accident', which is currently in vogue, is as non-specific as the term 'heart attack'. The cerebral vessels are branches of the internal carotid and vertebrobasilar arteries and are not subject to 'accidents': regional cerebral blood flow may be compromised by reduction in filling pressure, embolism, thrombosis or haemorrhage, causing symptoms and signs referable to a specific vascular territory, and should be diagnosed precisely whenever possible. The term 'stroke' is commonly used to describe any cerebrovascular event that causes a neurological disability.

Definitions

Transient ischaemic attack (TIA)

Neurological symptoms or signs lasting less than 24 h (usually 1–30 min).

Reversible ischaemic neurological deficit (RIND)

Symptoms or signs persisting more than 24 h but clearing over days or weeks.

Stroke

Permanent deficit from cerebral infarction or haemorrhage, which may be non-progressive (approximately 80%) or progressive (approximately 20%).

Prevalence

Approximately 14% of the population die of stroke, the third most common cause of death. TIAs occur as a warning in only 10–30% of stroke patients. Complete strokes are caused by thrombosis with or without embolism in 80% of cases, by cerebral haemorrhage in 10% and by subarachnoid haemorrhage in most of the remainder.

Pathogenesis

Most cerebral vascular disease is directly or indirectly attributable to atheroma. Factors included in the production of atheroma are:

Hypertension

Mortality from thrombotic and haemorrhagic stroke is twice as high in patients whose diastolic blood pressure is greater than 110 mmHg as it is in normotensive controls.

Hyperlipidaemia

Elevation of cholesterol and triglyceride levels is significantly associated with the onset of stroke under the age of 50 years.

Diabetes

Atheroma and stroke are more prevalent in diabetic patients.

Other factors contributing to TIA or stroke

Age

Cerebral vascular disease is more common with advancing years but may affect people in any decade of life.

Changes in the arterial wall

Atheroma   The extracranial vessels may be narrowed (stenosed) at their origin. The most common sites of stenoses are the bifurcation of the carotid artery, the origin of the vertebral arteries, and the basilar artery. These stenoses are common in people of middle or old age and are frequently symptomless; blood flow in the internal carotid artery is decreased only when the lumen is 2 mm² or less, and symptoms may then result if the blood pressure drops. The vessel may become completely occluded by thrombosis resulting in a cerebral infarction. Ulcers in an atheromatous plaque may be the site of platelet accumulation or the source of cholesterol crystals, either of which may embolize the distal cerebral circulation.

Arteritis Temporal arteritis may cause vascular occlusion in patients aged 55 years or older. Arteritis may also rarely be the cause of unexplained stroke in the first three decades of life. 'Moya moya' is a Japanese term (meaning mist, smoke or haze) used to describe the copious collateral circulation seen on angiography after occlusion of the distal part of the carotid siphon in young people. The collateral circulation fills the middle cerebral artery distal to the point of occlusion.

Rare causes of stroke These include fibromuscular hyperplasia, dissecting aneurysm of the arterial wall and direct trauma to the artery by a blow to the neck.

Sudden lowering of filling pressure

(a) Cardiac dysrhythmias or myocardial infarction with fall in cardiac output.
(b) Postural hypotension or a sudden fall in blood pressure from the use of hypotensive drugs.
(c) Blood loss or severe anaemia.
(d) Functional narrowing of extracranial portion of the arteries by neck turning.

Increased platelet aggregation or blood viscosity

(a) Polycythaemia vera.
(b) The use of oral contraceptive pills or other female hormonal preparations.
(c) Pregnancy, postpartum or postoperative states.
(d) The oligaemic phase of classical migraine (which is associated with increased platelet aggregation).

Forms of cerebral vascular disease

Transient ischaemic attacks

Carotid circulation (Figs 15.1, 15.2)

Approximately 50% of carotid TIAs are caused by thrombo-embolism from an atheromatous ulcer in the extracranial portion of the internal

Fig. 15.1 The vertebrobasilar and carotid arterial systems, showing their course in the neck and communication through the circle of Willis. (Modified from Lance, 1975, *Headache*, with permission of Charles Scribner's Sons, New York.)

carotid artery, usually at the bifurcation of the common carotid artery. Emboli consist of platelet and fibrin, or occasionally of cholesterol crystals, and can sometimes be seen passing through the retinal arteries during a TIA. The source of platelet emboli may also be intracranial, commonly at the carotid siphon or the origin of the anterior or middle cerebral arteries.

Less commonly, emboli may arise from atheromatous plaques in the aorta or from the heart in atrial fibrillation, from mural thrombi following myocardial infarction, and possibly from prolapsed mitral valves in young women. Septic thrombi from subacute bacterial endocarditis may lodge in distal branches of the cerebral vessels and produce mycotic aneurysms. Very rarely, fragments of atrial myxoma may embolize cerebral vessels.

Symptoms (a) Amaurosis fugax. Transient loss of vision in the ipsilateral eye, described as a curtain or shutter descending over the eye, caused by retinal embolization from a plaque in the internal carotid artery, is a symptom in 30% of carotid TIAs. Unilateral blindness may also be caused by insufficiency of the posterior ciliary artery supplying the optic nerve head (ischaemic papillopathy) (Fig. 9.7).

Fig. 15.2 Intracranial course of carotid and vertebrobasilar arterial systems. The basilar artery gives off the superior cerebellar arteries before terminating as the posterior cerebral arteries which supply the medial part of the temporal lobes and occipital cortex. The third cranial nerve emerges from the midbrain between the superior cerebellar and posterior cerebral arteries, close to the posterior communicating artery. (From Lance, 1975, *Headache*, with permission of Charles Scribner's Sons, New York.)

(b) Contralateral paraesthesiae or hemiparesis (each in 60% of cases).

(c) Transient dysphasia if the dominant hemisphere is involved (17% of cases).

(d) Headache, usually ipsilateral, in approximately 20% of cases.

Physical examination A harsh mid-systolic bruit may be audible at the angle of the mandible opposite the carotid bifurcation. A bruit may sometimes be heard on the side opposite the more severe stenosis because of increased blood flow on the relatively unaffected side.

Vertebrobasilar circulation (Figs 15.1, 15.2)

TIAs in vertebrobasilar territory are referred to as vertebrobasilar insufficiency (VBI) and, in contrast to carotid TIAs, are only rarely caused by thrombo-embolism from atheromatous plaques. Most cases appear to result from loss of normal autoregulation in the hindbrain circulation which leaves the patient vulnerable to any diminution of filling pressure.

An atheromatous plaque is sometimes found at the origin of one or both vertebral arteries. Particular attention must be paid to causes of hypotension as described above.

Two specific but rare causes of VBI should be sought.

Cervical spondylosis   Osteophytes project laterally from the neurocentral joints so that twisting of the neck may obliterate the lumen of the vertebral artery where it runs through the foramina transversaria of the cervical spine (Fig. 15.1).

Subclavian steal syndrome   Stenosis of one subclavian artery proximal to the origin of the vertebral artery may lower the filling pressure sufficiently to cause reversal of blood flow so that blood flows up the vertebral artery on the normal side and down the vertebral artery on the side of subclavian stenosis, thus 'stealing' blood away from the hindbrain circulation (Fig. 15.3). Symptoms of VBI may become apparent

Fig. 15.3 Subclavian steal syndrome. Stenosis of one subclavian artery converts the distal part of the artery (and the vertebral artery arising from it) into a low pressure system. Blood may thus flow up one vertebral artery and down the other, lowering basilar artery filling pressure and 'stealing' blood away from the brainstem to cause symptoms of vertebrobasilar insufficiency.

when the arm on the affected side is exercised, thus dilating the peripheral vascular bed and reducing pressure distal to the stenosis. Subclavian stenosis is not uncommon although the symptoms are rare. The condition is surgically remediable.

Symptoms of VBI

(a) Brainstem symptoms and signs. Vertigo (50% of cases), diplopia (40%), circumoral or unilateral paraesthesiae (40%), weakness of one or both sides of the body (33%) and falling or 'drop attacks' in 3% of cases (caused by ischaemia of the reticular formation).

(b) Cerebellar symptoms and signs. Dysarthria, ataxia or incoordination (33% of cases).

(c) Impairment of vision in one or both visual fields, i.e. right, left or bilateral homonymous hemianopia (from ischaemia of occipital cortex, supplied by posterior cerebral arteries which derive their blood supply from the basilar artery). Visual symptoms occur in about 60% of cases.

(d) There may be transient amnesia because the medial temporal lobe is also supplied by the posterior cerebral circulation.

(e) Occipital headache in about 20% of cases.

Physical examination

The radial pulses are asymmetrical in subclavian stenosis, the blood pressure being lower on the affected side. Blood pressure should always be taken in both arms of patients with VBI. A systolic bruit is usually heard above the clavicle over the site of the stenosis.

Prognosis of TIAs

Of patients with TIA, some 36% will suffer a complete stroke within 5 years, about half of these happening in the first year. Thereafter, the stroke rate is 5–6% per year (16 times that of control subjects who have never experienced TIAs). Ten year survival is 40%, compared with 60% for age-matched controls. It should be noted that death from myocardial infarction is twice as common as death from stroke. If hypertension is controlled, the mortality rate of patients with TIAs approximates that of normal controls.

Investigation of TIAs

All patients warrant a full blood count and ESR, as the ESR is greater than 40mm/h in two-thirds of patients with temporal arteritis. Other routine investigations comprise blood glucose, serum lipids, chest X-ray, electrocardiogram (plus echocardiogram if embolization from the heart is suspected). A CT scan of the brain will confirm cerebral infarction and haemorrhage and will help to exclude a cerebral tumour which may sometimes cause intermittent symptoms resembling those of TIAs.

Patients with unilateral carotid TIAs in general should be assessed by bilateral carotid angiography or four-vessel angiography, both performed by femoral catheterization. This demonstrates ulceration, stenosis or occlusion of extracranial and intracranial portions of the carotid circulation. Arteriography carries a risk of causing transient neurological deficit in 13% of such patients and permanent deficit in 0.65%. Angiography should therefore be carried out only if endarterectomy or some other surgical procedure is being considered, and it may be inadvisable in patients with evidence of generalized atheroma (angina, intermittent claudication).

Non-invasive methods of investigation include:
(a) Ultrasonic scanning of the carotid bifurcation ('real-time' B scanning gives a two-dimensional image adequate to detect some atheromatous plaques or ulcers).
(b) Ophthalmodynamometry. Measurement of the pressure at which retinal vessels cease to pulsate. A significantly low retinal arterial pressure indicates occlusion or gross stenosis of the internal carotid artery on that side.
(c) Directional Doppler flow studies may confirm the presence of internal carotid occlusion by detecting reversal of blood flow in the supraorbital artery on the affected side, since collateral circulation from the external carotid system feeds the internal carotid circulation by a retrograde flow in the ophthalmic artery.
(d) Regional cerebral blood flow studies by the inhalation of xenon-133, in centres where this technique is available.

Patients with VBI require an X-ray of the cervical spine and careful observation for postural hypotension or intermittent cardiac dysrhythmias (Holter monitoring of the ECG may be useful if attacks of VBI are recurring daily). Angiography is usually undertaken only if there is a localized bruit at the base of the neck or evidence of subclavian steal since the chance of showing a surgically correctable lesion is otherwise remote.

Present evidence in patients with an *asymptomatic carotid bruit* is that the risk of stroke is sufficiently low not to warrant angiography or endarterectomy. Some develop TIAs but the death rate is not much different from that of the general population — most deaths are from myocardial infarction and not from stroke.

Treatment of TIAs

General management

Hypertension, hyperlipidaemia and diabetes should be controlled in appropriate patients. It is advisable for patients not to smoke cigarettes or to use the contraceptive pill. Cardiac dysrhythmias, polycythaemia, anaemia or other underlying conditions should be controlled.

Specific management

Surgical Carotid endarterectomy in patients with unilateral disease appropriate to symptoms improves expectation of life as well as reducing risk of stroke. The combined mortality and morbidity rate of the procedure should not exceed 2%. In patients with disease of more than one vessel, operation may not improve the natural history of the disorder.

Bear in mind that life-expectancy depends on coronary rather than cerebral vessels. If coronary bypass surgery and carotid endarterectomy are both to be undertaken, results are better if the operation is done in two stages, the carotid surgery being done first. Either way there is a stroke rate of 3%, but this doubles if both procedures are done together.

Symptomatic subclavian steal syndrome is uncommon but is readily repaired surgically.

Operations on the cervical spine (removal of osteophytes or anterior interbody fusion) may rarely be indicated in some patients with VBI.

Anastomosis of the superficial temporal branch of the external carotid artery to the middle cerebral artery (EC/IC bypass) has been evaluated for the treatment of internal carotid and middle cerebral artery occlusion and found to be of no benefit in most cases.

Medical (a) Prevention of platelet aggregation in TIAs. Aspirin therapy (the optimal daily dose has yet to be determined) reduces the risk of stroke and death by one-third in males but not in females.

Sulphinpyrazone (Anturan) and dipyridamole (Persantin), other agents for preventing platelet aggregation, have not been proven to be useful in preventing stroke. Aspirin acts by irreversibly inhibiting the enzyme cyclo-oxygenase, thus preventing the formation of thromboxane A_2 from arachidonic acid for the life of the platelet (5–10 days).

(b) Anticoagulants. The administration of Warfarin to patients with TIAs with careful monitoring of prothrombin times, reduces the risk of stroke but does not reduce mortality since more patients die of cerebral haemorrhage and other conditions.

(c) Antispasmodics or vasodilators. These are of use *only* if the attacks are caused by migrainous vasospasm (migraine equivalents or transient migrainous accompaniments — TMAs), in which case the inhalation of isoprenaline spray as used for asthma, or oral administration of glyceryl trinitrate or nifedipine may be effective.

Cerebral infarction

The factors in the pathogenesis of cerebral infarction are the same as those discussed for TIAs as platelet aggregation can lead to thrombosis and infarction.

Since 90% of strokes occur without warning, the most effective long-term measure in prevention is the control of hypertension and hyper-lipidaemia at an early age, particularly in those people with a family history of cerebral vascular disease.

Clinical features

In 80% of cases, the patient presents with a completed stroke, the symptoms and signs of which depend upon the vascular territory affected. *Internal carotid occlusion* may be symptomless but commonly results in infarction in the ipsilateral hemisphere producing a contrala-teral hemiplegia, hemianaesthesia (and sometimes hemianopia) with the head and eyes turned to the side of the lesion, i.e. away from the hemiplegic side. Speech and other intellectual functions may be im-paired, depending on whether the dominant or non-dominant hemis-phere is infarcted. If infarction is extensive the patient may be obtunded or stuporose.

The symptoms of *middle cerebral artery occlusion* are much the same as described above. Flow in the ophthalmic artery may sometimes be impaired sufficiently by internal carotid occlusion to cause ipsilateral blindness. Obstruction of the distal branches of the *anterior cerebral artery* which supplies the 'leg area' of the cortex can cause a monoparesis of the contralateral leg, while occlusion of the recurrent branch of the anterior cerebral artery (Heubner's artery) infarcts the part of the internal cap-sule carrying descending motor pathways for movement of the lower face and arm on the opposite side of the body. Blockage of the parent trunk of the anterior cerebral causes hemiparesis by the combination of these effects.

A circumscribed infarction may result from occlusion of a small perforating vessel with localized brain softening and subsequent formation of a cyst or *lacune*. These usually occur in hypertensive patients. *Lacunar infarction* in the internal capsule or pons may cause a pure hemiplegia or, in the thalamus, may produce a pure hemianaesthesia which recovers in a few days. Some capsular or upper pontine lacunes may cause 'ataxic hemiparesis' in which weakness is accompanied by cerebellar signs on the same side because of involvement of corticopontocerebellar pathways. In hypertensive patients multiple lacunes can lead to pseudobulbar palsy (see p. 152).

Basilar artery occlusion causes brainstem infarction with bulbar palsy and quadriparesis so that the patient may be able to communicate only by eye movements ('locked-in syndrome') (p. 193). Various areas of the brainstem may be selectively infarcted by occlusion of the vertebral artery or branches of the basilar artery; for example, lateral medullary infarction from obstruction of the posterior inferior cerebellar artery or the vertebral artery which gives rise to it.

Homonymous hemianopia, cortical blindness and amnesia may also be features of basilar artery obstruction because the posterior cerebral arteries, which supply the medial part of the temporal lobes and the occipital lobes of the brain, arise from it (p. 153; Fig. 9.27).

Diffuse hypertensive cerebral vascular disease   In sustained hypertension the small perforating arteries of the brain may be obstructed, causing small areas of softening (lacunes), which may be symptomless or cause small strokes. When many such softenings develop bilaterally in the putamen, head of the caudate nucleus and internal capsule (*état lacunaire*), the signs of *pseudobulbar palsy* appear with bilateral spastic quadriparesis, upper motor neurone lesions of the lower cranial nerves, inappropriate and excessive laughter or crying, and dementia.

In 20% of cases, the stroke is not complete from the beginning but has a stuttering onset caused by the gradual occlusion of a major vessel, and is known as a 'progressive stroke' or 'stroke-in-evolution'.

Prognosis

If hemiplegia develops within 3 h and persists for 36 h there is a 90% chance that deficit will be permanent. Of patients with hemiplegia *and* impaired consciousness, 41% die. Of patients conscious on admission to hospital, more than 80% survive. Most patients can walk again and move the shoulder and elbow but not the hand. Unfortunately about one-third remain disabled and dependent.

Investigation

CT scan is the most useful investigation in completed stroke, since it distinguishes infarcts from haemorrhages. However, it does not invariably exclude subdural haematoma or some cerebral tumours.

Treatment

There is no evidence that the use of steroids, intravenous mannitol or dextran, sympathetic block, CO_2 inhalation or hyperbaric oxygen has any effect on a completed stroke. There is some evidence that intravenous mannitol may reduce mortality in the first week. The emphasis at present is on maintaining normal blood pressure, early rehabilitation and the prevention of a further stroke.

A progressive stroke may be treated by intravenous heparin but a CT scan should always be performed first since there is always difficulty in distinguishing a stroke-in-evolution from a TIA or a small cerebral haemorrhage.

Cerebral embolism

As discussed under the heading of TIAs, many strokes begin as cerebral emboli which may arise from the heart, carotid arteries or other great vessels.

The management is similar to that of cerebral thrombosis causing infarction. The underlying cause of embolism should be sought and treated; anticoagulant therapy may be indicated to prevent recurrence of emboli.

Cerebral haemorrhage

Intracerebral haemorrhage almost always occurs in hypertensive patients. Bleeding occurs from micro-aneurysms on small vessels (Charcot-Bouchard aneurysms). The blood clot may remain localized or it may infiltrate and destroy the surrounding brain. The most common sites are the putamen, thalamus, cerebellum and pons.

Clinical features

The onset may be rapid or gradual over a period of hours, often accompanied by headache. With the most common cerebral haemorrhage, that in the putamen and internal capsule, contralateral hemiplegia is the earliest symptom, followed by sensory loss, hemianopia and aphasia if the dominant hemisphere is affected. On examination there is usually a dense hemiplegia and the head and eyes are deviated away from the hemiplegic side. If bleeding continues the patient becomes drowsy and unconscious.

In pontine haemorrhage, the patient usually loses consciousness and dies within a matter of hours. In cerebellar haemorrhage, occipital headache, vertigo and vomiting usually occur at the onset.

Investigation

In cerebral haemorrhage the cerebrospinal fluid is blood-stained in about 90% of cases but CT scan of the brain is now most often employed to distinguish haemorrhage from infarction.

Management

Careful attention to the airway, oxygen therapy, care of bladder and skin, the use of intravenous or intragastric fluids, followed by physiotherapy, is the supportive treatment required for most patients. Patients with intracerebellar haemorrhages (10% of cases) require urgent surgical evacuation of the blood clot. Only occasionally is surgical treatment of value in the other cases of cerebral haemorrhage.

Subarachnoid haemorrhage (SAH)

Subarachnoid haemorrhage is haemorrhage into the subarachnoid space, the most common cause of which is a ruptured aneurysm of one of the major vessels at the base of the brain. Other causes of subarachnoid haemorrhage include angiomas, trauma, infections (mycotic aneurysms), and haemorrhage secondary to haemorrhagic diseases. The ratio of aneurysm to angioma as a cause of SAH in various Western series varies from 5:1 to 25:1, but in Asia angioma is a more common cause than aneurysm.

Clinical features

The most common symptoms of SAH are the sudden onset of headache, stiff neck, photophobia, vomiting and loss of consciousness. Pain in the back and legs may follow SAH after some days because of blood descending in the cerebrospinal fluid to irritate the cauda equina. On examination, the neck is usually rigid and Kernig's sign (p. 16) may be present. Cranial nerves, commonly the third nerve, may be compressed by an enlarging aneurysm of the internal carotid or posterior communicating arteries (see Figs 9.10 and 15.2 for anatomical relations) and focal neurological signs may be caused by rupture into the cerebral substance or by the extensive vasospasm which usually follows SAH. Subhyaloid haemorrhages are observed in the fundi in some 7% of patients and papilloedema in 13%. Fever, albuminuria, glycosuria, hypertension and ECG changes may be found in the acute phase. The possibility of spinal SAH must be considered if weakness has a paraplegic rather than hemiplegic distribution.

Investigation

A CT scan will usually show blood in the subarachnoid space or ventricles and may also demonstrate an aneurysm or angioma. A lumbar puncture may occasionally be required to confirm the presence of uniformly blood-stained cerebrospinal fluid (CSF). Xanthochromia of the supernatant CSF becomes apparent after 4–12 h and persists for at least 7–10 days after SAH. A lymphocytic cellular reaction and increase in CSF protein to 0.7–1.3 g/l usually follows SAH. If the patient is conscious, cerebral angiograms should be obtained as soon as possible. If the patient is obtunded, extensive vasospasm is likely to prevent the demonstration of any aneurysm so that angiography is best deferred until the patient's mental state improves.

Some 80% of aneurysms are found on the anterior (30%) and posterior (30%) communicating arteries or the middle cerebral artery near its division into branches within the Sylvian fissure (20%). If no aneurysm is shown by carotid angiography, the vertebrobasilar system should be demonstrated since 15% of aneurysms arise from the hindbrain circulation. Multiple aneurysms are found in 10–15% of cases.

Prognosis

About one-third of patients die with the first haemorrhage within 24 h, and of the survivors about one-third have a further SAH within the first four weeks if the aneurysm cannot be clipped surgically.

Management

Aneurysms should be operated on as soon as practicable after demonstration by angiography because of the danger of recurrent haemorrhage. If no aneurysm is demonstrated or surgery is not feasible, the patient is usually kept at rest in bed for several weeks with the room darkened as long as the photophobia persists. Epsilon aminocaproic acid, an antifibrinolytic agent, has been used to prevent re-bleeding by inhibiting lysis of the clot surrounding the aneurysm.

Unnecessary exertion should be avoided and the bowels kept loose by aperients to prevent straining during defaecation. The use of a bedside commode is usually preferable to the gymnastics required to use a traditional bedpan.

Carotico-cavernous fistula

Trauma, or rupture of a saccular aneurysm of the internal carotid artery within the cavernous sinus, may form a fistula that increases intra-orbital pressure with the development of a pulsating exophthalmos, periorbital oedema, conjunctival injection, ophthalmoplegia (because of involvement of nerves III, IV, and VI in the wall of the cavernous sinus; Fig. 9.12), pain around the eye and noises in the head and a carotid bruit. The fistula may be occluded by a balloon inserted by a catheter through the femoral artery and floated into place under angiographic monitor. Internal carotid blood flow is thus preserved.

Extradural haemorrhage

Extradural haemorrhage is usually caused by laceration of the middle meningeal artery by a fracture of the parietal or temporal bones. There is a history of head injury which may or may not be followed by a brief period of unconsciousness. Classically there is a lucid interval for some hours or even days after the injury before the patient becomes drowsy, usually with headache and vomiting. As the haematoma extends, consciousness is progressively impaired and the pupil on the side of the haematoma dilates because the third nerve is compressed in the tentorial notch by displacement downwards of the temporal lobe (p. 195). Urgent surgical treatment is required to evacuate the haematoma and prevent further bleeding. X-ray of the skull may show a fracture line but the diagnosis is most readily confirmed by CT scan of the brain. If the condition is advancing too rapidly for any investigation to be done, the placement of burr holes on the same side of the skull as the dilated pupil can be a life-saving procedure.

Subdural haematoma

Acute subdural haematoma

This presents after head injury in the same manner as an extradural haematoma and is dealt with in the same way.

Chronic subdural haematoma

This condition may develop slowly over days, weeks or months after a relatively minor head injury which tears one of the veins running from the cortex to a venous sinus. The head injury may be so trivial as to be forgotten, particularly if it took place during a bout of excessive alcohol intake. Subdural haematoma should be suspected in any patient with progressive impairment of intellect or memory, recent onset of headache or drowsiness or any other symptom suggestive of a space-occupying lesion. The diagnosis can usually be confirmed by a CT scan of the brain but, after some days, the density of the haematoma approaches that of the surrounding tissue, and it may escape detection. Radionuclide scan is usually positive in subdural haematomas of more than 3 weeks duration. If the index of suspicion remains high after CT and radionuclide studies are apparently normal, bilateral carotid angiography should be undertaken as the definitive investigation. It must be remembered that midline structures may not be displaced if subdural haematomas are bilateral. Once diagnosed, the haematomas are evacuated surgically.

References

Barnett H.J.M. (1979) The pathophysiology of transient cerebral ischaemic attacks. Therapy with platelet antiaggregants. *Med. Clin. North America* **63**, 649–79.

Harrison M.J.G. and Dyken M.L. (Eds) (1983) *Cerebral Vascular Disease. Neurology III.* Butterworths, London.

Ross Russell R.V. (Ed.) (1983) *Vascular Disease of the Central Nervous System*, 2nd edn. Churchill-Livingstone, Edinburgh.

Sloan M.A. (1987) Thrombolysis and stroke. Past and future. *Arch. Neurol.* **44**, 748–68.

Solomon R.A. and Fink M.E. (1987) Current strategies for the management of aneurysmal subarachnoid haemorrhage. *Arch. Neurol.* **44**, 769–74.

Swanson P.D., Calanchini P.R., Dyken M.L. *et al* (1977) A co-operative study of hospital frequency and character of transient ischemic attacks II. Performance of angiography among six centers. *J. Amer. Med. Ass.* **237**, 2202–6.

Toole J.F. (1984) *Cerebrovascular Disorders*, 3rd edn. Raven Press, New York.

Walton J.N. (1956) *Subarachnoid Haemorrhage.* Livingstone, Edinburgh and London.

Whisnant J.P., Cartlidge N.E.F. and Elveback L.R. (1978) Carotid and vertebral-basilar transient ischemic attacks: effects of anticoagulants, hypertension and cardiac disorders on survival and stroke occurrence — a population study. *Ann. Neurol.* **3**, 107–15.

16 Epilepsy

Epilepsy is a recurring disturbance of cerebral function caused by paroxysmal neuronal discharges, usually (but not always) accompanied by loss of consciousness. Attacks may consist of the sudden onset of sustained muscular contraction, producing an abnormal posture (tonic seizure), rhythmic jerking of the face, trunk or limbs (clonic seizure), or one phase followed by the other (tonic–clonic or *'grand mal'* seizure). Epilepsy may also take the form of a transient loss of consciousness (*petit mal* absence), a muscular jerk (myoclonus) or the sudden impairment of postural tonus, causing a falling attack (atonic or akinetic epilepsy). Some epileptic attacks, known as 'partial' or 'focal' seizures, reflect the function of the cortical area from which they arise and may be characterized by unilateral motor or sensory symptoms, or more complex states with hallucinations of the special senses and disturbances of memory or emotion ('complex partial seizures'), which usually originate in one temporal lobe.

Prevalence

Some 5% of children under the age of 6 years are liable to convulsions (tonic–clonic seizures) when body temperature becomes elevated, usually with an infection. These are known as 'febrile' or 'infantile' convulsions and, unless they cause severe hypoxia, have a good prognosis since only 10% of such children continue to have any form of epilepsy over the age of 6 years.

The prevalence of epilepsy in the community is generally estimated at 0.5% but the true prevalence is probably closer to 1%.

Classification

Epilepsy may be regarded as *symptomatic* or *idiopathic* depending on whether or not a cause (such as metabolic disturbance or a cortical lesion such as angioma or tumour) can be demonstrated.

The International Classification of Epileptic Seizures divides epilepsy into two main categories: *generalized epilepsy*, in which both hemispheres are involved virtually synchronously in the epileptic process; and *partial epilepsy*, in which the disturbance remains localized to one cortical area until the paroxysm ceases or becomes generalized.

Generalized epilepsy

Absences (petit mal)

An absence is a brief lapse of consciousness in which the patient, usually a child, stares blankly for a few seconds. The attack can be so transient that it may escape notice by patient and observer. It may be associated with any one or more of the following signs: fluttering of the eyelids, rolling upwards of the eyes, simple actions (automatism) such as fumbling with clothing, slight jerking of the limbs (myoclonus), passing urine, falling to the ground (akinetic attack).

The child who day-dreams, appears inattentive in class, or 'switches on and off' all the time should be suspected of having *petit mal* absences. The electroencephalogram (EEG) is very helpful in diagnosis, the characteristic abnormality being paroxysmal discharges of rhythmic 3 Hz spike-and-wave activity (Fig. 16.1). About 80% of children with absences lose their attacks by the end of the second decade of life.

Myoclonus

Myoclonus is jerking of the face, limbs or trunk, commonly affecting muscles asymmetrically, in which case it is usually made worse by voluntary movement (action myoclonus) or by sensory stimulation — a flash of light, sudden sound or touch (stimulus-sensitive myoclonus). A second variety is a rhythmic contraction of muscles which may cause symmetrical flexion of the limbs or trunk. This is usually seen in progressive cerebral disorders such as subacute sclerosing panencephalitis (SSPE) — a slow virus infection (see p. 266), or in infants with brain damage when the movements may become violent (infantile spasms). Rhythmic jerking of the palate (palatal myoclonus) may be seen in disease of the lower medulla but the term is misleading since it is a tremor rather than a manifestation of epilepsy.

Myoclonus is often seen in association with other forms of generalized epilepsy and a series of jerks may precede tonic–clonic seizures (*grand mal* fits). It may be of genetic origin in various forms of familial myoclonic epilepsy or may be acquired as the result of diffuse brain

Diffuse
thalamocortical
discharge

Fig. 16.1 3 Hz spike-wave discharge of generalized epilepsy, most commonly associated with *petit mal* absences. The paroxysms may arise in the reticular formation of the thalamus and midbrain as indicated, or may spread via associated fibres from one area of cortex to another. (From Lance and McLeod, 1981, with permission of Butterworths, London.)

damage such as hypoxia, encephalitis or metabolic disturbances. It is caused by a loss of normal inhibitory influences so that any afferent input to the nervous system leads to a synchronous motor response.

Akinetic attacks

An akinetic or atonic attack is a sudden unexpected fall, with or without loss of consciousness, caused by inhibition of the normal postural mechanisms. The *petit mal* absence is a temporary failure of the arousal mechanism responsible for consciousness, the upstream projection of the reticular formation (reticular activating system). The akinetic attack is a comparable disruption of the downstream projection of the reticular formation, the reticulospinal pathways. It is not surprising therefore that absences and akinetic attacks may occur together. The child who frequently falls without warning at home or in the school playground ('trips over his shadow') should be suspected of having akinetic attacks.

If absences and akinetic attacks are associated with tonic seizures and mental retardation (Lennox-Gastaut syndrome), the EEG usually shows atypical spike-wave paroxysms of 2–2.5 Hz and the prognosis for control of seizures is poor.

Infantile spasms (West's syndrome)   These are seizures, occurring in the first year of life, consisting of sudden muscle contractions. Character-istically, the child flexes forwards with outstretched arms ('salaam attacks'). The EEG is grossly abnormal ('hypsarrhythmia'). Most of these children are mentally retarded. The seizures may respond favour-ably to treatment with ACTH or corticosteroids.

Tonic–clonic seizures (major fits, grand mal *epilepsy)*

Before an attack, some patients have premonitory symptoms of elation, depression, irritability or headache. The classical epileptic seizure com-prises a tonic phase, in which facial, jaw, limb and trunk muscles contract, followed by a clonic phase with jerking of the limbs (Fig. 16.2). At the beginning of the tonic phase, which usually lasts for about 15–30s, patients may utter a cry as air is forced out of their lungs, bite their

Grand mal seizure

Fig. 16.2 Tonic–clonic seizure. The tonic phase, seen in muscle recordings (EMG), is associated with a high-frequency discharge in the EEG and reticular formation, which is later interrupted by inhibitory slow waves to give rise to EMG silent periods characteristic of the clonic phase. (From Lance and McLeod, 1981, with permission of Butterworths, London.)

tongue, then become cyanosed as apnoea continues in a position of forced expiration. The misguided insertion of a finger or firmer object into the mouth at the onset of the seizure serves only to amputate a phalanx or chip a tooth, each being a poor exchange for an unbitten tongue.

As the tonic phase passes into the clonic phase, patients may pass urine or occasionally open their bowels. The rhythmic jerking of the clonic phase gradually subsides, leaving patients in a state of stupor or confusion for some minutes or hours, after which they may complain of headache (or a painful back if a vertebral body or the paravertebral muscles have been injured during the tonic spasm).

If the seizure is preceded by focal neurological symptoms or signs (an 'aura'), these indicate a focal origin for the epileptic episodes with secondary spread to other cortical areas. The attack is then called a 'secondary generalized seizure' and attention is paid to the site of origin. A succession of tonic–clonic seizures, without the patient regaining consciousness, is known as 'status epilepticus'.

Partial (focal) epilepsy

The term 'partial' implies that the seizure involves a limited area of cortex and its thalamic connections (Fig. 16.3).

Fig. 16.3 Partial (focal) epilepsy. A potentially epileptic discharge may remain localized to one area of cortex or propagate via the corpus callosum to form a mirror focus in the opposite hemisphere. The discharge may spread over one or both hemispheres to produce a partial or generalized seizure. (From Lance and McLeod, 1981, with permission of Butterworths, London.)

Elementary (simple) partial seizures

Focal motor seizures   These attacks usually start with twitching of the face or thumb since the largest area of the motor cortex is devoted to control of facial and hand muscles. Rhythmic jerking may then extend down one side of the body as the epileptic 'march' progresses over the contra-lateral motor cortex (Jacksonian epilepsy, named after Hughlings Jackson, an English neurologist, 1835–1911, who made many contributions to the understanding of epilepsy).

Versive seizures   Turning of the head and eyes, usually to the side opposite an irritative lesion which is situated in the frontal eye-fields (area 8) or occasionally in the occipital lobe.

Focal sensory seizures   These may arise from the primary sensory cortex, causing contralateral paraesthesiae, or from the primary receptive areas for the special senses, causing unformed hallucinations of vision (flashes of light), or hallucinations of smell or hearing. Since the centres for smell and hearing are part of the temporal lobe, hallucinations derived from these areas are usually part of the syndrome known as 'complex partial seizures'.

Complex partial seizures

Seizures arising from the temporal lobe may include the following symptoms, associated with loss of consciousness.

Hallucinations of smell (olfactory) or taste (gustatory)   Such hallucinations are usually acrid or otherwise unpleasant, often associated with a 'dreamy state' (called *uncinate fits* by Hughlings Jackson because they arise from the region of the uncus in the anterior temporal lobe).

Hallucinations of hearing and vision   Abnormal sounds, such as buzzing, crackling or popping, or a transient sensation of movement (vertigo) may arise from the primary auditory receptive area in the superior temporal gyrus. More complicated hallucinations of conversation or music may originate in the auditory association cortex. Visions of animals, people or objects are derived from the visual association area or, rarely, a complete 'memory trace' combining visual, auditory and sometimes olfactory sensations may provide a 'play-back' of some past event.

Memory disturbances   Memory disturbances include transient amnesia, a false feeling of familiarity as though a place or conversation has been experienced previously (*déjà vu*) or the converse, the sensation of everything being strange and unfamiliar (*jamais vu*).

Illusions of time passing unduly rapidly or slowly
The rapid onset of emotions   Commonly an inexplicable ghostly fear, or more rarely an elevation of the mood to ecstasy, may arise from the temporal lobe. A child suddenly running to his or her mother in unreasoned terror should be suspected of having complex partial seizures.

Automatisms   The combination of impaired consciousness with the execution of relatively simple movements is known as an automatism. Automatisms may last up to 15 min and may consist merely of chewing movements, smacking of the lips and fumbling with objects but can be as intricate as driving a car through several sets of traffic lights without disaster.

Pathophysiology

Since most of us are subject to occasional *déjà vu* experiences or 'night starts' (resembling myoclonus) on drifting off to sleep, it is apparent that we all dwell on the rim of the epileptic volcano. Those who are engulfed by the eruption are victims of their genetic background, metabolic disturbances or some localized source of cortical irritation.

The epileptic neurone

The functional characteristics of neurones are altered in epilepsy so that dendrites are readily depolarized. Epileptic neurones may develop high frequency discharges because of failure of the normal modulation from surrounding cells, either as a result of gliosis or of diminution in inhibitory neurotransmitters. The repeated synchronous firing of epileptic neurones renders them more likely to discharge in the future, a phenomenon known as 'kindling'.

The spike-wave complex

Neurones are arranged radially with respect to the cortex, their dendrites ramifying in the superficial layer and their cell bodies lying deeply in layers 5 and 6 (Fig. 16.4). Waves of depolarization affect the dendrites, causing current flow from cell bodies to dendrites, which are recorded as negative spike discharges from the surface of the cortex or in scalp recordings (EEG). The spike discharge may be followed by a surface-

Fig. 16.4 Cortical origin of spike-wave discharge. Dendrites ramifying in superficial layers of the cortex are first depolarized so that current flows from the neutral cell body toward the cortex to form a surface-negative EEG spike. Following excitation of the neurone, the cell body becomes hyperpolarized by inhibition from recurrent fibres. Current thus flows from cell body to neutral dendrites, causing a negative slow wave in the EEG. (From Lance and McLeod, 1981, with permission of Butterworths, London.)

negative slow wave because, while dendrites recover from depolarization, their cell bodies become hyperpolarized as the result of inhibitory feedback circuits activated by the epileptic discharge (Fig. 16.4).

A spike-wave complex may therefore be recorded in the EEG from a localized abnormality in the cortex or may spread over the cortex through association fibres or to the opposite hemisphere via the corpus callosum. Such spread may cause a 'mirror focus' in the opposite hemisphere or cause generalized epilepsy without involving the reticular formation (Fig. 16.3).

The cause of generalized epilepsy

There is experimental evidence that *petit mal* absences may arise from the reticular formation of the midbrain and medial thalamus since they may be induced by stimulation of these central areas in young animals (Fig. 16.1). Major tonic–clonic seizures probably always arise from the cerebral cortex, either as spread from a focal cortical lesion or as a virtually simultaneous discharge throughout the cerebral cortex. Some forms of myoclonus, such as post-hypoxic myoclonus, are associated with deficiency in serotonergic transmission. Changes in other neurotransmitters such as gamma aminobutyric acid (GABA) have been postulated as factors in the causation of epilepsy.

Genetic factors

The 'spike-wave trait' is the genetic tendency to develop paroxysms of spike-wave complexes, usually at 3 Hz, which may not be associated with overt clinical seizures. It is inherited as a dominant characteristic, but fortunately clinical expression in the form of minor or major seizures is low. Some forms of temporal lobe epilepsy may be inherited by a dominant gene and some rare conditions such as progressive myoclonic epilepsy may be recessively inherited. There is also a family tendency to seizures, apart from any recognizable genetic pattern, to which many factors contribute.

Metabolic factors

Seizures may be caused, or their frequency increased, by: hypoxia; hypocapnia; hypoglycaemia; electrolyte disturbances, especially hypocalcaemia; fluid retention, e.g. at menstruation; hyperthermia; pyridoxine deficiency; withdrawal from sedative drugs or alcohol; drugs, heavy metals, insecticides, toxins; fatigue; pregnancy.

Local disturbances of cortical function

An epileptic focus may arise in an area of cortical gliosis or where part of the cortex has been isolated from its normal afferent inflow. Causes include the following:
(a) Cortical gliosis — birth trauma or hypoxia; head injury (the risk of epilepsy increases from 2% after a closed head injury to 40% in cases where the cortex is lacerated); meningitis, brain abscess, neurosyphilis.
(b) Sequel to prolonged febrile convulsions in childhood.
(c) Congenital abnormalities and inherited disorders — arteriovenous malformations (angiomas); hamartomas; tuberous sclerosis; cerebral lipidosis.
(d) Cerebral tumours, primary and secondary.
(e) Cerebral oedema (e.g. hypertensive encephalopathy).
(f) Vascular disease, cortical ischaemia or infarction.
(g) Cortical atrophy, e.g. the pre-senile dementia known as Alzheimer's disease.

Reflex precipitation of epilepsy

Some patients may have epilepsy induced by a specific form of afferent stimulation, the commonest being flickering light, e.g. on changing television channels ('television epilepsy').

Other rarer types of epilepsy are reading epilepsy and musicogenic epilepsy.

The investigation of epilepsy

When the patient is seen at the time of the first fit, life-threatening conditions such as hypoglycaemia and meningitis must be considered. It never does any harm to take a blood sample for glucose estimation and then to inject glucose intravenously in an unconscious patient; on some occasions it may be life-saving. Unless there are clinical signs suggestive of meningitis or subarachnoid haemorrhage, lumbar puncture is not usually necessary.

When the patient is seen in less urgent circumstances, the most useful diagnostic test is the EEG but it is a worthwhile routine to arrange a full blood count and ESR, blood glucose, calcium, electrolytes and serological tests for syphilis, as well as chest X-ray.

If the EEG demonstrates a diffuse spike-and-wave discharge, whether typical or atypical, the epilepsy is classified as generalized and the likelihood of a focal cerebral lesion is small, although focal lesions may sometimes be associated with secondary generalized discharges.

If the EEG shows a localized spike, sharp wave, or spike-and-wave discharge, it indicates a partial seizure originating from a focal cortical lesion, irrespective of the clinical manifestation of the seizure.

Any other EEG abnormality, such as asymmetry of normal rhythms, local or generalized slow activity, may indicate an underlying cerebral disturbance but is not specifically epileptogenic. A normal EEG does not exclude epilepsy. The record may remain normal even when some attacks, such as tonic seizures or some form of myoclonic jerking, are in progress.

If the clinical description of the attack or the nature of any EEG abnormality indicates a focal disturbance, further investigation is usually necessary, particularly in adults, to exclude cerebral tumour or other potentially remediable conditions.

Computerized axial tomography (CT scan) demonstrates most cerebral tumours and also shows the CSF pathways clearly so that it is the technique of choice for demonstrating hydrocephalus, a porencephalic cyst or cortical atrophy. It demonstrates acute extradural or subdural haematomas, but may miss subacute haematomas as the density of the haematoma then approaches that of the adjacent cerebral tissue. Areas of gliosis and small hamartomas are better demonstrated by magnetic resonance imaging (MRI) than by CT scanning.

Further investigations such as angiography may be required in some cases but these are the prerogative of a specialized neurological/neuro-surgical department.

A child or young adult in whom the clinical features and EEG suggest generalized epilepsy does not usually require any of the organ-imaging techniques since it is unlikely that they will contribute to diagnosis or management.

Management of epilepsy

The aim of managing epilepsy is to prevent the seizures entirely if possible so that the patient can lead a completely normal life. If the various metabolic and local causes of epilepsy have been excluded or if the family history and EEG indicate that the epilepsy is idiopathic then anticonvulsant medication can be started provided that the patient has had more than one seizure. Care must be taken that epileptiform movements during profound syncope are not mistaken for a primary epileptic disturbance. With present treatment about one-third of patients remain liable to seizures in spite of medication.

Psychological and social factors in management

It is important to place oneself in the position of a person who has previously been perfectly well and is suddenly told that he or she is suffering from epilepsy. Considerable time must be spent in explaining that many eminent people in the community have been subject to seizures but have succeeded in achieving their goals in their vocation and in their family lives.

Questions that commonly arise concern the following.

School

It is advisable for the child's school teacher and peer group to know the type of seizure to which the child is subject so that an attack does not lead to a panic reaction, and that reasonable supervision can be maintained. It is most important to ensure that an epileptic child is not singled out, teased or bullied by other children. The better educated the child, the more chance of his or her obtaining a suitable job later on, so that epilepsy should not be a reason for leaving school prematurely unless there is some associated condition such as mental retardation.

General activities

The patient should be encouraged to join in all normal activities with as few restrictions as possible. There are some common sense precautions to be taken. The patient should swim only in the company of some responsible person; a child should not climb trees to a great height or ride a bicycle on a busy road.

Driving

The current practice in most Australian states is that no one may hold a driving licence until 2 years have elapsed from the date of the last fit. Some exceptions are made; for example, a patient whose seizures have occurred only during sleep for a period of at least 2 years.

Occupation

The teaching and nursing professions, airlines, and the armed services do not usually accept anyone with a history of epilepsy. Julius Caesar, whose seizures before a battle were regarded as a good omen, would not be admitted to the ranks of a modern army. Any occupation that requires working at heights, electrical wiring or using moving machinery should be avoided. One of the professions or a trade or business in which the patient is self-employed gives the best opportunity for fulfilment.

General advice

Patients should be advised to avoid excessive fatigue, missing meals and taking more than the most modest amount of alcohol. There are many other questions that will arise, concerning marriage, having children and other life decisions which must be handled sympathetically with the knowledge of the particular patient and the most recent information available to guide the patient.

Anticonvulsant medication

Seizures can be controlled by medication in about two-thirds of patients. The appropriate drug must be selected and increased slowly to a dose which maintains a blood level in the therapeutic range without blunting the intellectual ability of the patient. Ideally, only one drug should be used (monotherapy), but if seizures are only partly controlled a second medication may be added. However, addition of a second drug benefits only about 15% of cases. The patient should understand the importance of taking medication regularly and continuing for at least 5 years from the date of the last seizure. Even then, if treatment is discontinued, 40% of patients will relapse and have further attacks.

Tonic–clonic and partial (focal) seizures

The most commonly used drugs for the control of major and focal (partial) seizures are phenytoin and carbamazepine, but a recent study has shown that sodium valproate is at least as effective as phenytoin in preventing major seizures when used as monotherapy.

Phenytoin (Dilantin)   Phenytoin is a hydantoin, first used for epilepsy in 1938. It is safe and effective but may cause coarsening of the features, excess body hair and swelling of the gums, particularly in children and adolescents. It is available as capsules of 100 mg and 30 mg, tablets of 100 mg and 50 mg, and a suspension for paediatric use of 6 mg/ml. The usual adult dose is 200–400 mg daily, given in divided doses twice daily, to maintain a blood level of 40–80 μmol/l. Dosage for children is estimated at approximately 10 mg/kg daily. The half-life is about 24 h. Overdosage causes nystagmus, dysarthria and ataxia. Phenytoin may cause a skin rash, lymphadenopathy and hepatomegaly as an idiosyncratic reaction. Long-term use may cause fall-out of Purkinje cells in the cerebellum.

Carbamazepine (Tegretol)   Carbamazepine is structurally related to tricyclic antidepressants and was introduced for the management of epilepsy in 1964. Tablets contain 200 mg or 100 mg carbamazepine, and the usual maintenance dose varies from 600 to 1200 mg daily, given in divided doses two or three times daily. Treatment is started with a low dose, e.g. 100 mg three times daily, since vertigo and ataxia are not uncommon initial side-effects. Leucopenia is common during carbamazepine therapy but rarely is severe enough to warrant cessation of treatment. Initially, the half-life of carbamazepine is 24–48 h, but this is reduced to about 9 h after continued use. The therapeutic range is 20–50 μmol/l.

Sodium valproate (Epilim, Depakine)   The anticonvulsant properties of sodium valproate were discovered in 1961 but it was introduced into general use only in the 1970s. It is effective in major and focal seizures and does not usually cause sedation. Since it is used also for *petit mal* absences and myoclonus, it is discussed under that heading.

Barbiturates   Phenobarbitone has been used as an anticonvulsant since 1912. It is cheap and effective but has the disadvantage of causing sedation and irritability in some patients, particularly children. The usual dosage varies from 90 to 300 mg/day to maintain a blood level of 45–75 μmol/l. It has a long half-life in adults of 3–4 days, and can therefore be taken as a single daily dose. Methylphenobarbitone (Prominal), which is broken down to phenobarbitone in the body, is given in double the dose of phenobarbitone but confers no special advantage. Primidone (Mysoline) breaks down to phenobarbitone and another metabolite, phenylethylmalonamide, in the body. It is probable that all three substances have an anticonvulsant action, so that primidone may be more effective than phenobarbitone although hard evidence is lacking. Dosage of primidone is usually 250 mg two or three times daily but a small dose is advisable to start with as it may cause vertigo when first used.

Clonazepam (Rivotril)   Clonazepam is one of the benzodiazepine series that has a more effective and sustained anticonvulsant action than diazepam (Valium), although both these drugs can be given intravenously in cases of status epilepticus. Clonazepam is useful for tonic–clonic, partial seizures and *petit mal* epilepsy but has the disadvantage that it may cause sedation, irritability and aggression. It is available as tablets of 0.5 mg and 2.0 mg, and the dose varies from 0.5 mg to 4.0 mg three times daily according to its clinical effect and the tolerance of the patient. It has a long half-life of about 20–40 h.

Petit mal *absences, myoclonus and akinetic attacks*

These 'minor' forms of generalized epilepsy are associated with a 3 Hz spike-wave pattern in the EEG and usually respond satisfactorily to treatment with sodium valproate or ethosuximide. However, it is advisable to use one of the anticonvulsants mentioned above in combination with ethosuximide since it has little action on major seizures, which may develop once the absences have been controlled. Troxidone (Tridione) has been withdrawn from the market because it caused severe leucopenia in some cases. Clonazepam can be used for resistant cases.

Sodium valproate (Epilim, Depakine)   Sodium valproate is available as 200 mg tablets, 500 mg enteric-coated tablets, and as a syrup for paediatric use containing 40 mg/ml. The usual starting dose is 200 mg morning and night, given after meals to minimize gastric irritation since the tablets liberate valproic acid in the stomach. The dose is slowly increased to 400 mg three times daily or even to double this dose if necessary. With doses of more than 1000 mg daily, the 500 mg enteric-coated tablets are more convenient to use than the smaller tablets. The drug has a short half-life in the plasma (6–9 h) so it is better given as three divided doses. It usually makes patients brighter rather than drowsier and may sometimes cause tremor and insomnia. It may increase appetite and cause weight gain. Prolongation of prothrombin time may be found but does not appear to be of clinical significance. Hepatic damage, fatal in some instances, has been reported, particularly in young children and when combined with other drugs. For this reason the drug should be stopped if there is continued nausea, weight loss or abnormal liver function tests. Like all newly introduced drugs, it should be used with caution but it can give satisfactory seizure control without sedation.

Ethosuximide (Zarontin)   Ethosuximide is used for the control of *petit mal* absences, 250 mg capsules being introduced twice daily and the dose then being increased to three or four capsules daily if necessary. It may cause drowsiness and bone marrow depression.

Status epilepticus

Diazepam, 5–10 mg, should be given intravenously over 2 min and repeated in 10 min if seizures persist. Intravenous therapy may be given continuously at the rate of 5–10 mg/h (50 mg in 500 ml saline). Side-effects are hypotension, bradycardia, and respiratory depression. Clonazepam (1–2 mg intravenously) may be more effective than diazepam in the treatment of status epilepticus.

Sodium amylobarbitone, 50–100 mg intravenously over 10 min, or phenobarbitone sodium, 200 mg by intramuscular injection, may be used if diazepam is ineffective, but these drugs produce respiratory depression and hypotension.

Slow intravenous infusion of 250 mg phenytoin in an adult who has been taking the drug, or of 1000 mg over several hours in an adult previously untreated, may help control seizures. Phenytoin is of no value if given intramuscularly. Regular anticonvulsant medication must be continued subsequently.

Paraldehyde (5–10 ml intramuscularly) is also useful if diazepam and phenytoin are not effective.

If other treatment is unsuccessful, general anaesthesia and muscle relaxants may be necessary. The important principle of management is to keep the patient well oxygenated at all times to prevent further cerebral damage.

Interaction between anticonvulsants

Sodium valproate increases blood levels of barbiturate. There are many possible interactions between anticonvulsants and it is sensible to obtain a new estimation of blood levels if a drug is added to or subtracted from the patient's medication.

Pregnancy

Anticonvulsant drugs do not appear to have a detrimental effect on the fetus when administered to the mother during pregnancy in most cases although the incidence of hare-lip and cleft palate is increased with phenytoin (Dilantin) therapy and some reports suggest that sodium valproate (Epilim) increases the likelihood of spina bifida. Discontinuing anticonvulsants and thus permitting seizures, or even status epilepticus, to occur presents a graver risk to the fetus than the continuation of a successful anticonvulsant regimen.

The surgical management of epilepsy

When a focal cerebral lesion has been demonstrated in a site consistent with the nature of the seizure and the EEG discharge, it may be removed surgically. Even if the causative lesion cannot be visualized by CT scanning or MRI, it may be localized by EEG techniques, sometimes involving intracerebral electrodes or recording at the time of operation (electrocorticography). Speech and memory are tested before operation by the intracarotid injection of amylobarbitone to determine hemisphere dominance for language and the ability to register memory in each half of the brain. The most common operation is anterior temporal lobectomy. Operation is usually reserved for patients not responding to anticonvulsant therapy.

References

Goldensohn E.S. (1977) The epilepsies. In *Scientific Approaches to Clinical Neurology*, pp. 654–92. Eds E.S. Goldensohn and S.H. Appel. Lea and Febiger, Philadelphia.

Eadie M.J. and Tyrer J.H. (1974) *Anticonvulsant Therapy. Pharmacological Basis and Practice*. Churchill-Livingstone, Edinburgh.

Lance J.W. and McLeod J.G. (1981) *A Physiological Approach to Clinical Neurology*, pp. 301–23. Butterworths, London.

Porter R.J. and Morsell P.L., Eds (1985) *The Epilepsies*. Butterworths, London.

Robb P. (Ed.) (1980) *Epilepsy Updated: Causes and Treatment*. Symposia Specialists, Miami.

Sutherland J.M. and Eadie M.J. (1980) *The Epilepsies. Modern Diagnosis and Treatment*, 3rd edn. Churchill-Livingstone, Edinburgh.

Turnbull D.M., Rawlins M.D., Weightman D. and Chadwick D.W. (1982) A comparison of phenytoin and valproate in previously untreated adult epileptic patients. *J. Neurol. Neurosurg. Psychiat.* **45**, 55–9.

17 Episodic Cerebral Symptoms (fits, faints and 'funny turns')

The present chapter deals with attacks that are not typically epileptic in nature but in which consciousness is impaired, postural control is lost or there is disordered perception of the body or its environment. The term 'spell', implying witchcraft, is still used in the USA for such episodes just as we speak of 'seizures', suggesting that the body has been seized by the devil. The magical element can be overcome by a little foreknowledge of the syndromes to be encountered.

Momentary loss of consciousness

Fit or faint? This is a common diagnostic problem. The diagnosis is made more difficult by the fact that some fainting attacks may cause a degree of cerebral hypoxia sufficient to trigger off epileptiform manifestations such as the eyes rolling upwards, stiffening of the limbs or clonic jerking of the limbs. If such attacks, clearly secondary to syncope, are labelled as epilepsy the misdiagnosis affects the victims' lives profoundly. It may alter their vocation, their approach to marriage and having children, their ability to hold a driving licence and may hamper their intellectual endeavours by unnecessary medication.

Fainting (syncope)

Fainting almost invariably occurs when the subject is standing or sitting upright and is preceded by symptoms of impending loss of consciousness — dimness of vision, a feeling of faintness, nausea and sweating.

Loss of consciousness can be forestalled by the patient lying down promptly. 'Putting the head between the knees' is a half-way measure that may or may not prove effective. There are two basic causes of syncope.

Failure of venous inflow to the heart

Common syncope ('vasovagal syncope')   This is caused by a loss of autonomic control of the splanchnic circulation, leading to a sudden drop in blood pressure, and vagal stimulation causing bradycardia. Syncope may follow prolonged standing, particularly on a hot day (church and the parade ground are favoured settings), or experiencing sudden pain or an emotional shock (the sight of blood, or having an injection).

Micturition syncope   During micturition the heart rate slows and may thus precipitate fainting in one whose blood pressure is already precariously poised after assuming the upright posture. The characteristic story is that the patient, usually a man because of the male custom of passing urine while standing, gets out of bed in the middle of the night for this purpose, feels faint while micturating and faints in the lavatory. No treatment is necessary other than advice about standing slowly after lying down or sleeping for any length of time, and sitting down to pass urine.

Cough syncope   This condition is caused by paroxysmal coughing which maintains a positive intrathoracic pressure long enough to impair venous return to the heart. The usual history is that a good club man, middle-aged and mildly atherosclerotic, tells a funny story at the bar with a cigarette in one hand and a drink in the other. Uncontrolled mirth leads to repetitive coughing until he slumps pulseless to the floor. The condition usually ceases once the patient stops smoking and learns to control both mirth and coughing while standing.

Postural (orthostatic) hypotension   Dizziness on standing from the lying or squatting position is not uncommon at any age, particularly in adolescents and the elderly, more so in hot weather when peripheral vessels are dilated. The symptoms are caused by a lag in constriction of splanchnic and peripheral vessels to maintain blood volume and hence blood pressure, and are best treated by graded exercise rather than medication. The tendency is increased after a debilitating illness, in anaemic patients or those with grossly dilated varicose veins which pool blood on standing.

Pathological conditions accompanied by orthostatic hypotension include *disorders of autonomic function* (Chapter 7): degenerative disorders of the central nervous system, such as idiopathic orthostatic hypotension, and the Shy-Drager syndrome in which there is progressive loss of the cells of origin of the preganglionic sympathetic efferent fibres in the intermediolateral columns of the spinal cord as well as degeneration of central tracts. There may therefore be pyramidal, extrapyramidal and cerebellar features in the Shy-Drager syndrome in addition to profound postural hypotension. Postural hypotension is also common in Parkinson's disease because of degenerative changes in the autonomic nervous system. Postural hypotension may be a symptom in some peripheral neuropathies, particularly the Guillain-Barré syndrome and those caused by diabetes and amyloid. In these conditions, fibres in the autonomic nervous system degenerate or demyelinate. Impotence, impaired sweating, and impaired bowel and bladder control may also be a feature of autonomic disorders.

Postural hypotension may result from *hyponatraemia* and *low blood volume* after overenthusiastic diuretic therapy or in Addison's disease. Low blood volume may also be the direct effect of blood loss. Postural symptoms may be a side-effect of treatment with hypotensive drugs, including beta-blockers, or with monoamine oxidase inhibitors.

Primary failure of cardiac output

(a) Paroxysmal cardiac dysrhythmias.
(b) Heart block of various types (Stokes-Adams attacks).
(c) Obstruction to outflow from the heart — aortic stenosis, mitral stenosis, atrial myxoma, ball-valve thrombus and primary pulmonary hypertension (the latter three are rare).

Management

The treatment of syncope is that of any causative lesion. Persistent postural hypotension may be treated with tight elastic stockings and a girdle to prevent pooling of blood in legs and lower abdomen, and drugs such as the mineral-retaining corticosteroid 9-alpha-fluorohydrocortisone (Fludrocortef), 0.1 mg two or three times daily. Dihydroergotamine, which constricts capacitance vessels, may also be helpful.

Epilepsy

Epilepsy may start as episodes of sudden loss of consciousness with or without warning symptoms, but without any of the characteristics of a tonic–clonic seizure. Any momentary prodromal symptom indicating a focal cortical origin is suggestive of epilepsy but longer-lasting non-specific symptoms such as dimness of vision and light-headedness favour a diagnosis of syncope. Syncope usually takes place when the patient is upright, but epilepsy can occur in the recumbent posture. Epilepsy may be followed by postictal confusion and headache, whereas a subject is usually clear-headed and well-orientated after a syncopal attack.

If there is absolutely no warning at all, the diagnosis lies between epilepsy and a sudden diminution of cardiac output (Stokes-Adams attacks).

Vertebrobasilar insufficiency

Since the vertebrobasilar system supplies the reticular formation of the brainstem and midbrain, sudden loss of consciousness may be a presenting symptom of vertebrobasilar insufficiency. In this case, the sudden onset of loss of vision, diplopia, circumoral paraesthesiae, vertigo or other symptoms derived from the hindbrain preceding loss of consciousness will give the clue to the diagnosis.

Falling attacks

Unexpected falls caused by the legs suddenly giving way without loss of consciousness may be of epileptic origin, usually in the younger patient (akinetic or atonic attacks).

The same symptom may occur in the older patient as a result of vertebrobasilar insufficiency, or at any age with a midline cerebral tumour such as a colloid cyst of the third ventricle. Apart from these clear-cut entities, falling attacks are not uncommon in middle age, affecting women more than men. Because their origin remains shrouded in mystery, they have been called 'cryptogenic falling attacks'. Careful history, examination and follow-up will usually determine that the falls are of either epileptic or vascular origin, or that there is an underlying cause such as polymyositis, multiple sclerosis, or other reason for intermittent weakness of the lower limbs.

Focal cerebral symptoms

Symptoms arising from various areas of the brain, cerebellum and brainstem have been described in earlier chapters. The clinical problem is to decide which of the following mechanisms is responsible in a patient presenting with an intermittent disturbance of a specific area of the brain.
(a) A fixed cerebral lesion such as angioma or tumour (or sometimes multiple sclerosis) causing intermittent symptoms by fluctuation in size or by surrounding cerebral oedema.
(b) Epilepsy, in which case a 'march of symptoms' from one cortical

area to another usually takes place over seconds or minutes, usually (but not always) preceding loss of consciousness.

(c) Migraine, when a similar 'march of symptoms' may take 10–60 min to complete, usually (but not always) preceding headache.

(d) Vascular insufficiency, usually characterized by a sudden onset of neurological deficit. It must be borne in mind that migrainous symptoms may develop in the atherosclerotic age group and thus be confused with thrombo-embolic episodes. These migrainous symptoms can usually be distinguished from thrombo-embolic episodes by the slow onset and resolution which is so characteristic of migraine. These late-onset migrainous equivalents have been called 'transient migrainous accompaniments' (TMAs) by Fisher (1980), to distinguish them from TIAs.

'Funny turns'

Hyperventilation (anxiety overbreathing)

This is one of the most common syndromes encountered in clinical practice and is frequently overlooked in the search for some sinister disease. Overbreathing may take the form of:

(a) Occasional deep sighing respirations or yawning (often accompanied by air swallowing). (b) Subclinical overbreathing. Each breath is just a little deeper than required, indicating an anxiety state to the shrewd observer. (c) Panting respiration, which is obvious even to an untrained observer

Overbreathing causes hypocapnia, with resulting cerebral vasoconstriction and diminution in ionized calcium, which is responsible for the following symptoms.

Mild hyperventilation

A constant sensation of light-headedness or dizziness; the sensation of instability on walking; dryness of the mouth; distension of the upper abdomen with excessive belching or passage of flatus (from associated air swallowing).

Moderate hyperventilation

Faintness, blurred vision; increasing anxiety; increase in heart rate; tightness in the chest; tingling of face and hands; coldness and sweating of the hands; headache.

Severe hyperventilation

Crushing sensation in the chest; a feeling of panic or impending death; tremor or shaking with a jelly-like feeling in the legs as though the patient might collapse; spasms of the hands and feet (carpo-pedal spasm), a form of tetany from deficient ionized calcium.

Precipitating factors

Symptoms are often worse when the patient is in a crowd, e.g. a cocktail or dinner party, shopping in a crowded street or supermarket (agoraphobia).

Management

The first step is to convince the patient of the diagnosis since many suspect that they have asthma, angina pectoris, epilepsy or labyrinthine vertigo. One of the commonest causes of giddiness in practice is anxiety overbreathing. The patient must be taught to watch for the signs of overbreathing, especially sighing, yawning or tightness in the chest and then to hold the breath deliberately for 10 s before breathing out slowly, then to regulate the respiration at no more than 10 breaths/min. The underlying anxiety state should be handled by psychological advice and by relaxant or antidepressant drugs if necessary. A course of relaxation training is helpful. General advice about not hurrying unnecessarily, not bottling up anxiety or resentment and not smoking excessively, not drinking more than six cups of tea or coffee each day or missing meals will set a more relaxed pace which is less likely to produce symptoms of anxiety.

Breath-holding attacks

Breath-holding attacks are usually the prerogative of infants or young children as a dramatic expression of their discontent — usually rage or frustration. They may become cyanosed (or less commonly pale, generally after a head injury), lose consciousness and have minor clonic jerkings of the limbs. Theories of management differ from time to time but calm reassurance and soothing of the infant and parents usually has the desired effect although the child must remain subject to normal discipline so that he or she will not employ the attacks to manipulate domestic situations.

Toxi-confusional states

Metabolic disturbances such as hypoglycaemia, uraemia, hepatic encephalopathy and inappropriate secretion of antidiuretic hormone (ADH) may cause a fluctuating confusional state. Overdosage with bromides, lithium, barbiturates, anticholinergics, anticonvulsants or other drugs may have the same effect.

Excessive sympathetic activity

Acute anxiety state

This has been considered under the hyperventilation syndrome. Sympathetic activity and noradrenaline secretion are expressed as tremor, increased heart rate and excessive sweating.

Phaeochromocytoma

Symptoms include sustained or episodic hypertension and sudden attacks consisting of headaches (in 80%), pallor, tremor, sweating and palpitations. The diagnosis is confirmed by the estimation of catecholamines in at least three 24-hour specimens of urine, one collection of which should follow a typical attack. The tumour may lie anywhere along the sympathetic chain from neck to scrotum but the majority are in the adrenal area and can be localized by CT scan of the abdomen.

Temporal lobe epilepsy

This may produce the sudden sensation of fear associated with anxiety symptoms. The onset is rapid, the attack brief and often associated with *déjà vu* or other symptoms of temporal lobe discharge.

Hypoglycaemia

Catecholamine secretion is increased by hypoglycaemia since catecholamines induce gluconeogenesis which tends to restore the blood glucose levels to normal. Thus, tremor, sweating, pallor and palpitations may accompany mental confusion in hypoglycaemia.

Causes of hypoglycaemia are as follows:
(a) Iatrogenic — insulin administration; oral hypoglycaemic agents.
(b) Spontaneous — hyperfunction of pancreatic beta cells, insulinoma or hyperplasia; reactive to glucose intake, either functional, postgastrectomy, or a result of diabetes; sensitivity to leucine, to galactose in infants

and to alcohol in adults; liver disease; non-pancreatic neoplasms, e.g. retroperitoneal or intrathoracic fibrosarcoma; glycogen storage disease; endocrine disorders, such as hypopituitarism, Addison's disease, adreno-genital syndrome, pluriglandular syndrome.

Narcolepsy

Narcolepsy is a sudden irresistible desire to sleep which may come on many times during the day, often in inappropriate situations such as the school classroom or an important board meeting, as well as travelling on trains or buses. Sleep usually lasts for 10–15 min, after which the patient awakens refreshed. The condition must be distinguished fom the day-time somnolence associated with sleep apnoea. Narcolepsy, which is linked with HLA-DR2, may be associated with the following.

Cataplexy

Physical weakness on emotion such as laughter or rage. The patient may slump in his seat or even collapse to the ground after hearing a funny story or losing his temper. It is an extension of the normal sensation of feeling 'weak with laughter'.

Sleep paralysis

Complete inability to move or speak lasting for minutes usually coming on at a time of relaxation such as drifting off to sleep or awakening from sleep. The attack ceases spontaneously or on afferent stimulation, e.g. if someone touches the patient.

Hallucinations

These also occur on going to sleep (hypnogogic hallucinations) or on awakening from sleep (hypnopompic hallucinations). They usually consist of ghostly figures seen by the bedside.

All of these manifestations are an exaggeration of normal experiences, probably caused as a release phenomenon from the arousal system of the reticular formation.

Narcolepsy usually responds to methylphenidate (Ritalin) or amphetamines while cataplexy is most readily controlled by imipramine (Tofranil).

Movement disorders

Odd movements such as those of focal epilepsy and paroxysmal choreoathetosis have been considered in the appropriate chapters, as have causes of episodic muscular paralysis like hypokalaemia.

Hysteria

Hysteria may mimic any of these transient cerebral disturbances but some fits initially thought to be hysterical because of their bizarre nature have later been shown to be accompanied by temporal spike discharges so caution is advised in diagnosis.

The general message to be absorbed from a study of unusual episodic syndromes is that there are many organic causes and that one should not leap to the conclusion that any strange disorder which one has not seen before is necessarily of hysterical origin.

Reference

Fisher C.M. (1980) Late-life migraine accompaniments as a cause of unexplained transient ischemic attacks. *Canad. J. Neurol. Sci.* **7**, 9–17.

18 Cerebrospinal Fluid

The chief functions of the cerebrospinal fluid (CSF) are to:
(a) provide physical support for the brain and spinal cord.
(b) act as a vehicle for the excretion of waste products of brain metabolism.
(c) control the chemical environment of the central nervous system.
(d) enable intracerebral transport of chemicals and hormones, e.g. hypothalamic releasing factors.

Anatomy and physiology

The total volume of the CSF is approximately 150 ml, of which 75 ml are in the intracranial cavities. The ventricular volume of the CSF is only about 16 ml of which 7 ml are in each lateral ventricle, 1 ml in the third ventricle and 1 ml in the fourth ventricle.

Formation

The CSF is mainly formed and secreted by the choroid plexus of the cerebral ventricles, but there is also evidence for extrachoroidal formation in the brain and spinal cord with transependymal secretion. The CSF formed in the lateral ventricles flows into the third ventricle through the interventricular foramina and then through the aqueduct into the fourth ventricle to reach the subarachnoid space by way of the foramen of Magendie and the foramina of Luschka. In this space it fills the cerebral cisterns, flows down and back up again in the spinal subarachnoid space, and passes upwards over the convexity of the cerebral hemispheres (Fig. 18.1). The rate of CSF formation is relatively constant at 500 ml/day (0.35 ml/min).

Fig. 18.1 The circulation of CSF. CSF is formed in the choroid plexuses in the lateral ventricles (LV), third ventricle (3) and fourth ventricle (4), passing out from the ventricular system through the foramina of Magendie and Luschka to pass over the hemisphere in the subarachnoid space and to be absorbed in the arachnoid villi. (From Lance, 1975, *Headache*, by permission of Charles Scribner's Sons, New York.)

Absorption

Most of the reabsorption of CSF is through the arachnoid villi in the intracranial venous sinuses but there is also some absorption in the spinal canal adjacent to the spinal roots. The rate of absorption, within broad limits, is directly related to the CSF pressure. The blood–brain barrier is maintained by tight junctions of capillary endothelial cells, choroidal epithelium and arachnoid membranes. In some regions such as the area postrema, parts of the hypothalamus and subfornical and subcommisural organs, the barrier does not exist.

The blood–brain barrier can be altered by pathological states including anoxia, ischaemia, toxins, infections and some endocrine disorders.

Characteristics

Adults and older children

Glucose: 2.9–4.6 mmol/l
Protein: Ventricular 0.05–0.15 g/l
          Cisternal   0.15–0.25 g/l
          Lumbar   0.15–0.40 g/l (0.15–0.30 g/l) in children
          IgG   0.07–0.38 g/l (5–12% of total protein) in adults
                        0.07–0.17 g/l (3.5–8.7% of total protein) in children
Cells: 0–4×10^6 cells/l (normally lymphocytes/monocytes)

Pressure: 65–195 mm CSF (5–15 mmHg)

Newborns

The CSF protein is high at first (up to 1.2 g/l) and gradually drops to childhood levels by about 3 months of age. The white cell count is also elevated in the newborn — up to about 20×10^6 cells/l being common, often with a predominance of polymorphs. Xanthochromia is also common in the neonate.

Lumbar puncture

Because the spinal cord normally ends at about the level of the first lumbar vertebra, a needle can be inserted into the spinal subarachnoid space below this level without fear of cord injury.

Indications

(a) Diagnosis of diseases. The main value of CSF examination is to diagnose *meningeal inflammation* (Chapter 19) or *bleeding* (Chapter 15) into the subarachnoid space. Although changes in the CSF occur in other diseases (e.g. tumours and vascular disease) the changes are often non-specific and a diagnosis can often be reached with more accuracy and safety by other means.

(b) Introduction of therapeutic agents or local anaesthetics into the subarachnoid space.

(c) Introduction of diagnostic agents into the subarachnoid space, e.g. contrast media such as metrizamide for myelography and CT scanning, radio-isotopes for ventriculocisternography, and air for pneumo-encephalography.

(d) Measurement of CSF pressure. This should rarely be the sole indication for lumbar puncture, except in neurosurgical hands (see contraindications below). However, the CSF pressure must always be measured whenever a lumbar puncture is performed.

(e) Therapy. Regular lumbar puncture has been employed as a means of reducing CSF pressure in benign intracranial hypertension.

Contra-indications

The presence of papilloedema is an absolute contra-indication to lumbar puncture until a CT scan has excluded a space-occupying lesion, and suspicion of raised intracranial pressure is a relative contra-indication to the procedure. Thus, a lumbar puncture should not be done primarily to see if the pressure is raised. The danger of lumbar puncture in the presence of raised intracranial pressure is that withdrawal of fluid may cause herniation of the medulla through the foramen magnum ('coning') leading to medullary compression and death. In supratentorial space-occupying lesions, herniation of the medial temporal lobe may occur through the tentorial opening which results in compression of the midbrain and possible death (uncal herniation) (Chapter 13). The mortality of lumbar puncture in cerebral abscess is appreciable.

Infection of the skin in the lumbar region near the site of puncture is also a contra-indication.

Complications

(a) Headache, caused by reduced pressure. The treatment is to have the patient lie flat with the foot of the bed elevated and drink copious fluids.

(b) Pressure coning — see above.

(c) Damage of a nerve root, which is usually caused by placing the needle too far laterally.

(d) Infection. When usual sterile precautions are taken, this is very uncommon.

(e) Transient back stiffness.

Abnormalities of CSF

Naked eye appearance

CSF is normally clear and colourless.

Turbidity

This is due to excessive numbers of cells, usually polymorphs, e.g. meningitis.

Blood

Presence of blood may be due to either traumatic tap or subarachnoid haemorrhage. In a traumatic tap the CSF is most heavily stained at the beginning and then usually gradually clears. In a subarachnoid bleed it remains evenly blood-stained. If the CSF is collected in three separate tubes ('the three tube test'), in a traumatic tap the fluid usually appears clearer in the third tube than in the first.

Xanthochromia

The presence or absence of xanthochromia (yellow colouration) after the fluid has been centrifuged is the most valuable method of distinguishing a subarachnoid bleed from a traumatic tap. Xanthochromia appears about 4 h after a subarachnoid bleed and reaches a maximum after about 36 h and gradually disappears over 7–10 days. It is due to the presence of oxyhaemoglobin, bilirubin and methaemoglobin.

Cells

The cell count normally does not exceed 4×10^6 cells/l, all mononuclear.

Polymorphs

Polymorphs usually indicate an acute inflammation, e.g. acute bacterial or viral meningitis. However, they may also appear after chemical irritation (e.g. myelography, air encephalography) or with trauma, haemorrhage or infarction.

Mononuclear cells

Mononuclear cells are increased in viral infections, chronic inflammations (e.g. tuberculous, fungal, carcinomatous meningitides), demyelination, cerebral infarction and some other conditions.

Protein

A mild or moderate rise in protein up to about 0.8 g/l is common but non-specific since it occurs in many disease states. High protein levels (over 1.0 g/l) are seen most commonly in spinal cord tumour causing obstruction of the subarachnoid space, meningitis, haemorrhage, demyelinating polyneuritis and some brain tumours.

Immunoglobulins

The CSF IgG is normally about 5–12% of the total CSF protein. It is increased in a number of conditions, but has particular diagnostic value in multiple sclerosis. In clinically definite multiple sclerosis it is raised in about 80–90% of cases. The ratio of IgG to albumin in the CSF can be measured and is usually less than 25%. Discrete oligoclonal bands of IgG may be demonstrated on electrophoresis in about 90% of patients with clinically definite multiple sclerosis.

Glucose

Glucose content is very low or absent in pyogenic meningitis and moderately low in chronic meningitides (e.g. tuberculous, fungal, carcinomatous). The level is high in diabetes mellitus, paralleling the blood glucose. When an abnormality in CSF glucose is suspected it should be compared with a blood glucose level taken simultaneously with the CSF; it is normally 60–80% of the blood glucose level.

Serological tests for syphilis

The most commonly employed screening tests are the reagin tests (e.g. VDRL). Positive reagin tests in the CSF are virtually diagnostic of neurosyphilis, although false positives may occur if there is a 'bloody tap'. The tests may remain positive when disease is inactive.

Hydrocephalus

Hydrocephalus is an increase in the volume of CSF associated with dilatation of the cerebral ventricles.

Causes

Obstruction

Intraventricular (non-communicating hydrocephalus)   The obstruction is within the ventricular system and may be at the foramen of Monro, third ventricle, aqueduct, fourth ventricle, or foramina of Luschka and Magendie due to neoplasms, congenital defects and inflammatory lesions such as meningitis. Mumps and possibly other intra-uterine infections may cause aqueduct stenosis.

Extraventricular (communicating hydrocephalus)   There is a free communication of the ventricular system with the subarachnoid space. This type of hydrocephalus may result from adhesions of the subarachnoid spaces at the base of the brain following infections or haemorrhage. Other causes include congenital defects such as the *Arnold-Chiari malformation* (a tongue of cerebellar tissue with an elongated medulla protruding into the spinal canal) or developmental absorptive defects of the arachnoid villi.

Defective absorption

Impaired venous sinus drainage may be caused by lateral or sagittal sinus thrombosis, or congenital or acquired (e.g. inflammation, high CSF protein) defects of the arachnoid villi. The lateral sinus may thrombose as a complication of mastoiditis (*otitic hydrocephalus*).

Overproduction

This is known to occur only in the very rare condition of choroid plexus papilloma.

Aetiology and pathology

The most common type of congenital hydrocephalus is that associated with the other major congenital abnormalities of meningomyelocoele and encephalocoele. Hydrocephalus is associated with 80% of cases of myelomeningocoele. It is due either to aqueduct obstruction or to associated Arnold-Chiari malformation. In occasional cases, intra-uterine infection (toxoplasmosis, cytomegalovirus infection and syphilis) is the aetiological factor. Rare cases have a genetic basis (X-linked recessive).

The aqueduct is the most common site of obstruction in congenital hydrocephalus; it may be congenitally abnormal (e.g. forked) or simply of very small calibre (aqueduct stenosis). There is ventricular enlargement, proximal to the site of block. The cerebral white matter is greatly thinned whereas the grey matter of the cerebral cortex is preserved until late in the course of the disease.

Clinical features

In congenital hydrocephalus developing in infancy the most common symptoms and signs are: head enlargement; delayed motor skills; pyramidal tract signs in the lower limbs due to stretching of corticospinal fibres (those destined for the lower limbs have a long course around the lateral ventricles from their origin on the medial side of the hemisphere and are thus most liable to damage); and optic atrophy, which is a late complication of chronic papilloedema due to increased intracranial pressure.

In older children and adults with acquired lesions there are symptoms of raised intracranial pressure such as headaches, nausea, vomiting and diplopia.

Diagnostic studies

Head measurement   The circumference of the head should be compared with normal values on a standard head-size chart (Fig. 2.1). Serial measurements showing a crossing of percentiles are very important. Increased head size may also be caused by megalencephaly (brain of excessive size and weight), bone abnormalities (e.g. achondroplasia and rickets), chronic subdural haematoma in infancy and some other rare conditions.

Transillumination of the head   A torch is applied to the baby's head in a dark room. Abnormal redness around the torch indicates an excessive amount of fluid beneath the torch, e.g. hydrocephalus, subdural effusion, localized cerebral cysts.

Skull X-ray   A large head and widened sutures may be seen in a child with hydrocephalus. The sutures can widen with raised intracranial pressure until the age of about 10 years. In older children and adults, after the cranial sutures have fused, the signs of raised intracranial pressure are erosion of the dorsum sellae and clinoid processes.

Neuroradiology   CT and MRI scans, pneumoencephalography and ventriculography will demonstrate enlarged ventricles and possibly the site of obstruction.

Echo-encephalography   This is a useful non-traumatic investigation for diagnosing and following the size of the lateral ventricles in children under the age of about 4 years.

Treatment

Removal of the primary lesion neurosurgically if possible (e.g. posterior fossa tumour); or insertion of a shunt.

A variety of methods for diverting CSF flow have been devised. The current popular methods are the ventriculo-atrial and ventriculo-peritoneal shunts using non-reactive tubing and pressure valves.

Unfortunately complications of shunts occur, and these include blockage causing raised intracranial pressure, infection, pulmonary emboli with ventriculo-atrial shunts, and shunt nephritis, an immunologically determined disorder due to secondary *Staphylococcus albus* infection.

Normal pressure hydrocephalus

Normal pressure hydrocephalus is a syndrome of adults characterized by insidious onset of memory and intellect impairment, which progresses to a severe dementia with an apraxia of gait and urinary incontinence. Headache is not a feature and there are no signs of raised intracranial pressure; there is no papilloedema and CSF pressure is normal.

There is marked ventricular dilatation present on CT scan without evidence of cortical atrophy. These findings are in contrast to those in cerebral atrophy where the sulci are very prominent and secondary ventricular enlargement occurs (hydrocephalus *ex vacuo*). Normal pressure hydrocephalus is, in fact, a communicating hydrocephalus with obliteration of the subarachnoid space over the surface of the cerebral hemispheres. It may be secondary to subarachnoid haemorrhage, meningitis, or trauma or may occur spontaneously. The CSF pressure is said to be normal or low (hence the term normal pressure hydrocephalus). The continuous monitoring of intracranial pressure through an intraventricular catheter shows that rises of pressure to abnormally high levels occur at times, particularly during sleep. Isotope cisternography is helpful in the diagnosis. This investigation consists of introducing a radio-isotope into the CSF and then performing radionuclide scanning to observe its flow. In normal pressure hydrocephalus the radio-isotope remains in the ventricular system and does not appear in the subarachnoid space over the surface of the brain.

About 50% of patients with normal pressure hydrocephalus respond well to surgical shunting procedures.

Benign intracranial hypertension (pseudotumour cerebri)

Benign intracranial hypertension is a condition in which increased intracranial pressure occurs in the absence of a space-occupying lesion or obstruction to CSF flow, and with normal or small ventricular size.

Aetiology and pathology

In most adults the cause is unknown but it is most commonly seen in obese young females and presumably has an endocrine basis. It may be secondary to a thrombosis of one or more of the dural sinuses, particularly the lateral sinus as a sequel to otitis or mastoiditis (otitic hydrocephalus). Benign intracranial hypertension may follow withdrawal of corticosteroids, Vitamin A intoxication, tetracycline and nalidixic acid administration.

Clinical features

The symptoms are those of raised intracranial pressure: headache, vomiting, blurred vision and diplopia due to an abducens nerve palsy (a false localizing sign). Papilloedema is almost invariably present. In contrast to raised intracranial pressure secondary to an expanding lesion, the patient looks well and has a normal level of consciousness and normal intellectual function.

Apart from the signs due to raised intracranial pressure, there are no other abnormal neurological findings.

Diagnosis

Investigations to exclude a space-occupying lesion must be undertaken and a diagnosis of benign intracranial hypertension cannot be made until these are all demonstrated to be normal. On CT or MRI scan there are no space-occupying lesions visible and the ventricles are normal or small in size.

Prognosis

Although the disease is often self-limiting, treatment of intracranial hypertension is necessary in order to prevent blindness occurring as a result of chronic papilloedema which may lead to secondary optic atrophy.

Treatment

The raised intracranial pressure may be reduced with corticosteroid therapy. Other forms of treatment such as acetazolamide and other diuretics and repeated lumbar puncture are also employed. Ventricular shunting procedures may be necessary, particularly the insertion of a shunt from the spinal subarachnoid space to the peritoneum (lumbar-peritoneal shunt).

Reference

Fishman R.A. (1980) *Cerebrospinal Fluid in Diseases of the Nervous System.* W.B. Saunders, Philadelphia.

19 Infections of the Central Nervous System

The chief infections of the nervous system are meningitis, encephalitis and abscess.

Meningitis is inflammation of the meninges. It may be classified as *purulent* or *pyogenic (i.e. meningitis due to bacterial infections), fungal*, or *aseptic* (most commonly due to viral infections but sometimes caused by chemicals, physical agents, parasites and malignant infiltration).

Encephalitis is inflammation of the brain substance itself. It is often accompanied by inflammation of the meninges (*meningo-encephalitis*). *Acute disseminated encephalomyelitis* is a diffuse demyelination of the brain and spinal cord which is usually an immune reaction following infections such as mumps, influenza, chicken pox, rubella, vaccinations or other injections (p. 227).

Meningitis

Acute bacterial meningitis

Infections may reach the meninges through the bloodstream or by direct spread from the middle ear and paranasal sinuses or through skull fractures.

The most common organisms causing meningitis are *Neisseria meningitidis* (meningococcus), *Streptococcus pneumoniae* (pneumococcus), and *Haemophilus influenzae*. In the neonatal period Gram-negative organisms (e.g. *E.coli, Proteus, Pseudomonas*) and Group B streptococci are common causative organisms. *Haemophilus influenzae* meningitis occurs in infants predominantly, whereas infection by pneumococcus and meningococcus may occur at all ages. In immunosuppressed patients, less common organisms such as *Listeria monocytogenes* may be responsible.

Pathology

The fundamental process is an inflammation of the leptomeninges with hyperaemia of the meningeal vessels, followed by migration of neutrophils into the subarachnoid space. The exudate rapidly extends into the walls of blood vessels and along cranial and spinal nerves. Foci of necrosis develop in walls of veins and arteries, sometimes leading to thrombosis which may be manifested clinically by convulsions and focal neurological signs. Accumulation of fibrino-purulent exudate at the base of the brain may block the flow of CSF causing hydrocephalus. Loculation of infection to form abscesses may be a further complication.

Clinical features

In adults the signs and symptoms are fever, headache, neck stiffness, nausea, vomiting, drowsiness, confusion and sometimes convulsions. Neck stiffness is a cardinal sign in adults and older children, but it may be absent in infants and neonates in whom the main clinical features are irritability, lethargy, feeding difficulties, vomiting, respiratory distress and fever. Focal neurological signs are usually absent unless complications develop.

Complications include acute hydrocephalus, with herniation of the brainstem and temporal lobes through the tentorial notch, or of the cerebellum and medulla through the foramen magnum (Chapter 13); thromboses of venous sinuses or cortical vessels causing seizures, hemiplegia and other focal neurological signs; cranial nerve palsies and deafness; subdural effusion; communicating hydrocephalus due to adhesions at the base of the brain or non-communicating hydrocephalus from obstruction of the aqueduct of Sylvius or foramina of Luschka and Magendie.

Management

Lumbar puncture with examination of the CSF is essential for diagnosis and should be carried out without delay when meningitis is suspected. Blood cultures should be performed, and sources of infection should be carefully sought in ears (otitis media), paranasal sinuses, heart (bacterial endocarditis), lungs, and skin.

Treatment consists of:

(a) Antibacterial chemotherapy. Initially, therapy should be administered intravenously. When the organism is unknown treatment in adults is commenced with ampicillin (12–18 g/day) or chloramphenicol (4–6 g/day). In children, empirical treatment is commenced with ampicillin (200 mg/kg per day) and chloramphenicol (75–100 mg/kg per day). More recently, with the emergence of penicillin resistant strains of *H. influenzae*, cefotaxime (200 mg/kg per day) has been used. Specific treatment subsequently depends on the results of culturing the causative organism in the CSF.

(b) Supportive measures — general nursing care, attention to airways, reduction of fever, hydration and maintenance of fluid and electrolyte balance.

(c) Treatment of complications if they occur, e.g. seizures, hydrocephalus, abscess.

Tuberculous meningitis

The onset is usually gradual with non-specific symptoms of lethargy and headaches followed by mental confusion. Later complications include seizures and arteritis causing focal neurological signs. Diagnosis depends on the clinical features and CSF findings, although commonly the organism is not cultured. Treatment is specific chemotherapy, i.e. isoniazid (400 mg/day), rifampicin (600 mg/day), ethambutol (1.5 g/day) and pyrazinamide (25 mg/kg per day).

Fungal infections

Fungal infections may also cause a chronic meningitis with an insidious onset and clinical features similar to those of tuberculous meningitis. The most common organism is *Cryptococcus neoformans*. Others include *Candida, Aspergillus* and *Histoplasma*. Most cases of fungal infection of the nervous system occur in immunosuppressed patients and in those with lymphoma, leukaemia and other malignancies, but they may present in otherwise healthy patients. Diagnosis is made on lumbar puncture by the characteristic appearances of the CSF and by culturing the organism.

Cryptococcal meningitis is treated with amphotericin B and 5-fluorocytosine.

Parasitic infections

Amoebic meningo-encephalitis is most commonly caused by *Naegleria*, and the infection is usually acquired while swimming in freshwater lakes. The onset is acute with headache, fever and neck stiffness.

Toxoplasmosis causes meningo-encephalitis and brain abscesses usually in patients with AIDS, malignancies, or in those who are receiving immunosuppressive therapy.

The nematode *Angiostrongylus cantonensis* causes an acute eosinophilic meningitis. It is well recognized in Southern Pacific regions and is acquired by eating freshwater snails and raw vegetables that have been contaminated by the parasite.

Carcinomatous meningitis

Metastatic spread of carcinoma to the leptomeninges causes a chronic meningeal reaction or meningitis which must be distinguished from infections of the meninges. The CSF contains increased lymphocytes, elevated protein and frequently a reduced glucose level. Malignant cells may be recognized in the fluid.

Viral (aseptic) meningitis

The clinical features of viral meningitis are similar to those of bacterial meningitis. The CSF contains lymphocytes, but few if any polymorphs and the glucose level is normal whereas it is usually markedly decreased in bacterial and fungal meningitis.

The distinctive features of the CSF in the different types of meningitis are shown in Table 19.1.

Usually the causative virus is not determined, but the most common causes of viral meningitis are ECHO, coxsackie, mumps, herpes simplex and measles. The polio virus can cause an aseptic meningitis but fortunately poliomyelitis is now rare.

Encephalitis

Encephalitis is usually caused by a viral infection of the brain and is associated commonly with aseptic meningitis. The main clinical features are headaches, fever, delirium, convulsions and focal neurological signs. Herpes simplex, mumps, and arboviruses are the most commonly identified organisms.

Herpes simplex encephalitis

Herpes simplex encephalitis is caused by the herpes simplex virus (HSV), usually type 1, and is one of the most common sporadic viral infections of the central nervous system. The virus enters the nervous system by way of the olfactory bulb, or a latent infection in the trigeminal ganglion may be reactivated and spread to the brain through its branches innervating the meninges. The pathology is that of a focal necrotizing encephalitis localized predominantly in the temporal lobes. Although the onset may be acute, symptoms of headache, fever, mental confusion and epileptic seizures usually evolve over several days. Examination of the CSF reveals an increased number of cells, mainly lymphocytes, and increased protein content. HSV antibodies may be detected but are of little diagnostic value since they may be present in

Table 19.1   CSF in infections of the nervous system

	Cells	Protein	Glucose	Bacteriology
Normal	0–4 mononuclears	0.15–0.40 g/l	2.9–4.6 mmol/l	Negative
Acute bacterial meningitis	Thousands of polymorphs	Increased	Markedly decreased	+ Bacteria
Partially treated bacterial meningitis	Hundreds to thousands of mononuclears or polymorphs	N or increased	N or decreased	+ or −
Aseptic meningitis	Tens to hundreds of mono-nuclears**	N or increased	N*	Viruses
Meningo-encephalitis	Tens to hundreds of mononuclears	N or increased	N*	Negative or viruses
Tuberculous meningitis	Tens to hundreds of mononuclears	Increased	Decreased	+ Acid-fast bacilli
Fungal meningitis	Tens to hundreds of mononuclears	Increased	Decreased	+ Organism
Carcinomatous meningitis	Tens to hundreds	Increased	N or decreased	Malignant cells
Neurosyphilis (meningo-vascular, syphilitic meningitis, GPI)	Tens to hundreds of mononuclears	Increased. Raised gamma-globulins	N*	+ Serological tests
SSPE	N	Increased. Raised gamma-globulin	N	Very high measles antibody titres
Creutzfeldt-Jakob disease	N	N	N	N
PML	N	N	N	N

* Glucose may be low in herpes simplex and mumps virus infections, and acute syphilitic meningitis.
** Polymorphonuclears may predominate in early illness.
N normal.
GPI general paralysis of the insane.

anyone who has had a previous HSV infection. EEG and CT scan characteristically demonstrate abnormalities in one or both temporal lobes. Mortality is high and can be significantly reduced by early treatment with acyclovir (30 mg/kg per day, intravenously).

Herpes zoster

The herpes zoster-varicella virus invades and lies latent in sensory ganglia. When reactivated, the symptoms of herpes zoster (shingles) are manifested by pain, a vesicular eruption and loss of sensation in distribution of the particular nerve root. Nearby motor nerves may sometimes be involved causing localized muscle weakness and wasting. Thoracic and trigeminal nerve roots are most commonly affected. When the first division of the trigeminal nerve is involved (*herpes ophthalmicus*) corneal ulceration and iritis may result in blindness. The *Ramsay-Hunt syndrome* consists of a unilateral facial palsy with herpetic eruptions in the external auditory meatus and is thought to be due to viral invasion of the geniculate ganglion although the pathogenesis is controversial. The pain of acute herpes zoster responds well to steroids or acyclovir but there is no evidence that the incidence of post-herpetic neuralgia is reduced after a course of one or both agents.

Arbovirus encephalitis

Arboviruses are arthropod-born viruses which are spread by mosquitoes. The best known are equine encephalitis and St Louis encephalitis in the United States, and Japanese B encephalitis, Ross River and Murray Valley encephalitis in Australia. The clinical features are headache, drowsiness, vomiting, convulsions and frequent focal neurological signs which may be permanent. There is no specific treatment.

Subacute sclerosing panencephalitis (SSPE)

SSPE is caused by the measles virus and affects children and adolescents, evolving over some months. Early symptoms are mental and behavioural changes followed by myoclonic jerks. Death usually occurs within 1–2 years. The EEG shows characteristic periodic complexes which may be diagnostic. The CSF cell content is not increased but the protein is elevated with high gamma globulin levels and high titres of measles virus antibodies. There is no specific treatment.

Creutzfeldt-Jakob disease

This is caused by a transmissible slow virus and has similarities to kuru and scrapie. It usually presents in middle age as a rapidly progressive dementia associated with ataxia and myoclonic jerks. Like SSPE, there is a characteristic EEG abnormality consisting of periodic complexes. The CSF is normal. Death usually occurs within 1–2 years and there is no specific treatment.

Progressive multifocal leukoencephalopathy (PML)

This is caused by the SV40 or JC papova viruses and occurs mainly in patients with lymphoproliferative diseases and other disorders associated with disturbed immunity. There are progressive multifocal lesions in the white matter.

Acquired immunodeficiency syndrome (AIDS)

The neurological manifestations of human immunodeficiency virus type 1 (HIV-1) infection result from direct invasion of the brain by the retrovirus or from opportunistic infections.

An important complication resulting from direct invasion of the brain is the *AIDS-dementia complex* which occurs in over 30% of AIDS patients. There is progressive mental confusion, intellectual deterioration, slowing of motor function and hyper-reflexia. Other manifestations of direct viral invasion include: vacuolar myelopathy, the symptoms of which are leg weakness and paraesthesiae, ataxia and incontinence; acute or chronic inflammatory polyneuropathy; and aseptic meningitis.

The most common opportunistic infections are toxoplasmosis, cryptococcal meningitis and progressive multifocal leukoencephalopathy. Zidovudine (azidothymidine; AZT) suppresses replication of HIV and prolongs life in AIDS patients. It is expensive and frequently suppresses bone marrow function. It is presently indicated for patients who have had one episode of *P. carinii* pneumonia or for patients with advanced AIDS-related complex.

Neurosyphilis

The central nervous system is usually invaded within 2 years after the primary infection, if at all. The principal types of neurosyphilis are acute syphilitis meningitis, meningovascular syphilis, general paralysis of the insane, and tabes dorsalis.

Acute syphilitic meningitis

Meningeal involvement usually takes place within the first 2 years of disease. Most cases are asymptomatic but others present with the typical symptoms of acute meningitis, i.e. headache, mental confusion and neck stiffness. The CSF contains an increased number of lymphocytes (100–1000 cells/mm³), elevated protein, reduced glucose and positive serological tests for syphilis.

Meningovascular syphilis

This develops about 6–7 years after the primary infection. As well as meningeal inflammation there is vasculitis with thrombotic occlusions of blood vessels. The clinical manifestations are those of cerebrovascular disease; neurosyphilis should be considered in the differential diagnosis of young people with strokes. The CSF shows increased lymphocytes, raised protein and gamma globulin, and positive serology. Spinal syphilis and syphilitic optic atrophy are specific complications of chronic syphilitic meningitis.

General paralysis of the insane

This complication usually develops about 15–20 years after the primary infection and is characterized by dementia, dysarthria, tremor, epileptic seizures, pyramidal tract signs, and sometimes Argyll Robertson pupils. The CSF is abnormal with increased lymphocytes (50–200 cells/mm³), increased protein and gamma globulin, and positive serological tests.

Tabes dorsalis (p. 105)

Treatment

Procaine penicillin 600,000 Units, intramuscular injection, daily for 15 days. If the patient is sensitive to penicillin, oral tetracycline (0.5 g six-hourly for 30 days) should be prescribed.

Brain abscess

Brain abscesses occur (i) as complications of penetrating head wounds; (ii) following extension of infections from the middle ear or paranasal sinuses; (iii) following bloodstream infection, frequently in association with cyanotic cogenital heart disease, bacterial endocarditis and pulmonary infections.

Initially, the infection commences as an inflammation of the brain parenchyma (cerebritis) with oedema, and is followed by necrosis in the centre of the lesion with pus formation. Headache, fever, lethargy, seizures and focal neurological signs are the usual presenting symptoms. The brain abscess acts as an expanding lesion causing raised intracranial pressure and papilloedema. Lumbar puncture should never be performed when an abscess is suspected. Most abscesses are visible on CT or radionuclide scans.

Treatment is antibiotic therapy; neurosurgery may be required later. Abscess has a high mortality rate and epilepsy is a complication in over 50% of survivors. Abscesses, as well as forming within the brain substance, may collect in the subdural space (subdural empyema) or in the spinal epidural space (spinal epidural abscess).

References

Johnson R.T. (1982) *Viral Infections of the Nervous System*. Raven Press, New York.

Johnson R.T. and Warren K.S. (1986) Parasitic infections. In *Diseases of the Nervous System*, pp. 1394–1405. Eds A.K. Asbury, G.M. McKhann and W.I. McDonald. W.B. Saunders, Philadelphia.

Sugar A.M. and Diamond R.D. (1986) Fungal infections. In *Diseases of the Nervous System*, pp. 1406–15. Eds A.K. Asbury, G.M. McKhann and W.I. McDonald. W.B. Saunders, Philadelphia.

Wood M.J. and Geddes A.M. (1987) Antiviral therapy. *Lancet* **2**, 1189–93.

20 Demyelinating Diseases of the Central Nervous System

Demyelinating diseases of the central nervous system are characterized by foci of degeneration of the myelin sheath around nerve fibres in the white matter of the central nervous system. The axon may also be damaged but the primary pathological process involves destruction of myelin.

Multiple sclerosis is the most common and important of these conditions but other demyelinating diseases include acute disseminated encephalomyelitis, neuromyelitis optica (Devic's disease) and diffuse sclerosis (Schilder's disease).

Multiple sclerosis

Multiple sclerosis is a disease which affects mainly people in the younger age groups and, in its most common form, is characterized by relapses and remissions. The lesions are disseminated in both space (different parts of the central nervous system white matter) and time (new foci of demyelination occur at intervals over a period of many years).

Aetiology

Although the cause of multiple sclerosis remains unknown, it is clear that both environmental and genetic factors are involved. The environmental factor may be a virus infection in childhood, the virus then possibly lying dormant in the nervous system until some later date when, because of a genetically determined defect in the immune mechanisms, central nervous system demyelination occurs.

The chief evidence for an environmental agent is epidemiological. The frequency of multiple sclerosis is related to latitude; there is a higher prevalence in temperate climates than in tropical and subtropical climates. In Australia the prevalence increases from 11.8 per 100 000 population in tropical Queensland to 75.6 per 100 000 in Hobart, Tasmania (Fig. 20.1). Migration studies indicate that a subject moving from

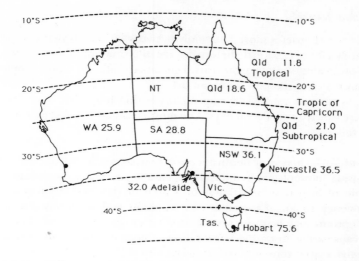

Fig. 20.1 Prevalence of multiple sclerosis in Australia. Standardized prevalence expressed as number of cases per 100 000 population at 30 June, 1981.

a high risk to a low risk zone in adult life has a greater chance of later developing multiple sclerosis than someone migrating as a child. This observation indicates that critical exposure to the environmental factors occurs in early years of life.

There is familial incidence of multiple sclerosis; approximately 10% of patients have an affected relative. However, the chief evidence for genetic influences is the strong association of the disease with the HLA system. In Caucasian races, there is an association with HLA-A3, HLA-D7 and HLA-DW2. Over 60% of patients are HLA-DW2 positive compared with only 15–20% of controls.

Pathology

The acute lesion is a perivenular infiltration of lymphocytes, macrophages and plasma cells associated with demyelination. In the later stages glial proliferation occurs; some axons are lost and only a very limited degree of remyelination occurs. The gliotic areas form discrete grey coloured areas within the white matter and are termed plaques. Plaques of demyelination occur predominantly in the white matter of the periventricular regions of the cerebral hemispheres, subpial regions of the spinal cord and the optic nerves.

Clinical features

The age of onset is most commonly between 20 and 50 years. Approximately 20% of cases arise before the age of 20 but only about 2–3% have an onset after the age of 50 years. Females are affected more commonly than males in the ratio of about 2:1.

Symptoms usually develop rapidly within hours but may develop more slowly over several days. The most common initial symptoms are as follows.

Weakness   There may be abrupt onset of weakness in one or more limbs causing monoplegia, hemiplegia or paraplegia. The patient may complain of heaviness or stiffness of a limb or tiredness, weakness or a tendency to fall. Fatiguability is common and weakness and other symptoms may be more pronounced in hot weather or after hot baths because a rise in temperature causes a block in conduction across the demyelinated zone in affected nerve fibres.

Optic neuritis (pp. 120–1)   Acute optic neuritis is a common early symptom. The vision becomes blurred and sight may be lost completely in one eye. There may be associated pain on eye movement and on pressure applied to the eye. The vision usually improves over a few days to weeks, and normal vision may return although there is commonly some residual impairment of colour vision. If the lesion lies near the optic disc, swelling of the disc may be observed on ophthalmoscopic examination but, if the lesion is more posteriorly placed in the optic nerve, no abnormality will be seen. On plotting the central fields of vision a central or paracentral scotoma is usually present and this can be more readily detected with a red target. Optic atrophy with pallor of the disc, especially in the temporal part, may be a sequel to optic neuritis. Permanent blindness is rare. Visual evoked potentials, which enable the conduction of the visual pathways to be assessed neurophysiologically, are abnormal in about 90% of patients with clinically definite multiple sclerosis even though they may give no history of optic neuritis.

Sensory symptoms   Numbness of one or more limbs or of the face is common in multiple sclerosis. A lesion in the dorsal columns may cause sensations of apparent swelling of the limbs or feelings similar to tight bandages or strings being wrapped around the limb. A band-like sensation around the waist may develop. A plaque in the cervical cord may cause a sensation resembling an electric shock down the back on flexing the spine (Lhermitte's sign). A clumsy or useless hand may result from a lesion that involves a dorsal root entry zone and dorsal columns by impairing proprioception. Trigeminal neuralgia may sometimes be caused by demyelination.

Unsteadiness of gait Ataxia of gait due to weakness, proprioceptive disturbance or cerebellar dysfunction is common.

Double vision Brainstem lesions may cause double vision by involvement of the ocular motor pathways. Internuclear ophthalmoplegia, due to a lesion in the medial longitudinal fasciculus, is a common cause of diplopia in multiple sclerosis (pp. 130–1).

Vertigo Vertigo may be an early symptom of multiple sclerosis and results from a brainstem lesion involving the vestibular pathways and the pons.

Sphincter disturbances Frequency, urgency and precipitancy of micturition or retention of urine may be initial symptoms of multiple sclerosis and sphincter disturbances are very common in later stages of the disease. Impotence frequently occurs.

Mental changes Mental changes are rarely initial symptoms of multiple sclerosis but are found later in the disease. Emotional instability, depression and euphoria are common.

Precipitating and aggravating factors

There are a number of factors which are considered but not proven to precipitate attacks of multiple sclerosis. They include infections, trauma, surgical operations, pregnancy, emotional stress, exertion and fatigue, and vaccinations and inoculations. There is a slightly increased risk of exacerbation occurring during pregnancy or after delivery but there is no evidence that this makes any difference to the long-term course or prognosis of the disease. Vaccinations and inoculations may precipitate relapse and should be avoided if possible; emotional stress is difficult to evaluate objectively but there is no firm scientific evidence that it influences the course of multiple sclerosis.

Clinical course and prognosis

About 80% of patients have a relapsing and remitting course and in a proportion of these the disease may subsequently become progressive. The remaining 20% have a progressive course from the outset. The chronic progressive form tends to have a later age of onset and a worse prognosis. About 10% of patients die within 15 years but the mean survival is 30 years. Guides to a poor prognosis are a late onset, a short interval between the first two relapses and the onset of a progressive phase of the disease.

Diagnosis

The clinical diagnosis of multiple sclerosis depends upon evidence from the history and examination of lesions in the central nervous system at more than one site and various episodes of involvement separated by an interval of time. According to the degree of certainty of the diagnosis, it may be classified as clinically 'definite', 'probable' or 'possible'. In taking the history it is important to ask about any previous neurological symptoms, such as blurring or loss of vision, numbness, tingling, weakness, double vision and sphincter disturbances. Occasionally symptoms are paroxysmal in nature, e.g. episodes of ataxia, or dysarthria of short duration. Tic douloureux and Bell's palsy may also be manifestations of multiple sclerosis. On physical examination it is important to look carefully for more than one site of involvement, e.g. if the patient has spastic paraparesis explicable by a single spinal cord lesion, examine carefully for evidence of cranial nerve involvement, such as optic atrophy and nystagmus. If all the symptoms and signs can be explained by a lesion at one site in the nervous system, multiple sclerosis should not be diagnosed and every effort should be made to exclude by appropriate investigations other causes, such as a tumour.

Certain diagnostic tests may be of value in confirming the diagnosis.

CSF

Cells   The cell count is normal (less than 3–4 lymphocytes/mm^3) in 60–70% of patients in remission. However, during relapse about 60% of patients have an increased cell count. The cell count rarely exceeds 50 cells/mm^3.

Protein   The total CSF protein is raised in only about 30% of patients with multiple sclerosis and it is exceptional for the value to be greater than 1.0 g/l.

Gamma globulin   The gamma globulin tends to be elevated in patients with multiple sclerosis. The ratio IgG/albumin in the CSF is normally less than about 25% and it is increased in approximately 60% of patients with clinically definite multiple sclerosis. IgG index compares the IgG/albumin ratio in the CSF and blood and is abnormal in about 90% of patients with clinically definite multiple sclerosis.

Oligoclonal bands   Oligoclonal IgG may be detected by agarose gel electrophoresis of the CSF or by isoelectric focusing. The latter technique is more sensitive but has a higher incidence of false positive results. Abnormalities are detected in about 90% of patients with clinically definite multiple sclerosis.

Electrophysiological studies (pp. 312–4)

The *visual evoked response* is a means of testing conduction in the visual pathways. The stimulus to the retina is usually that of a moving chequerboard pattern and the potential from the visual cortex is recorded through scalp electrodes (Fig. 20.2). The potential is delayed or reduced in amplitude in the presence of demyelinating lesions in the optic pathway and is abnormal in about 90% of patients with clinically definite multiple sclerosis.

Somatosensory evoked potentials may be recorded through scalp electrodes over the sensory cortex or from over the cervical spine on stimulating sensory nerves in the arms or legs. They are abnormal in about 70% of patients with clinically definite multiple sclerosis.

Auditory or *brainstem evoked potentials* can be recorded through surface electrodes after click stimuli are applied to the ears. They are abnormal in about 50% of patients with clinically definite multiple sclerosis and abnormalities indicate a lesion in the brainstem.

Fig. 20.2 Visual evoked potential recorded from a normal subject. Major positive peak (P100) has a latency of 92 m/s.

One or more evoked potentials are abnormal in over 90% of patients with clinically definite multiple sclerosis. The techniques are valuable in detecting clinically silent lesions and they therefore enable lesions in unsuspected sites to be diagnosed. The electrophysiological abnormalities persist; very rarely do they return to normal.

The CT scan

The CT scan may sometimes reveal plaques of demyelination but the yield of abnormalities is relatively low.

Magnetic resonance imaging (MRI)

Plaques and periventricular demyelination in the brain are readily demonstrated in over 90% of patients with clinically definite multiple sclerosis. The lesions are more difficult to demonstrate in the spinal cord, but the yield has been increased by use of the contrast agent gadolinium.

Treatment

There is no specific treatment for multiple sclerosis. Short courses, in reducing doses over four weeks, of ACTH and corticosteroids have been shown to be effective in shortening the duration of acute exacerbations, but they have no effect on the long-term course or prognosis of the disease. A number of forms of treatment have been aimed at reducing the severity or rate of progression of the disease but no form of treatment has been shown to cure or even stop the progression of multiple sclerosis. Extensive trials of different forms of immunotherapy have been undertaken, including prednisone, azathioprine, cyclosphosphamide and anti-lymphocyte globulin may slow down the rate of progression of the disease, but all have serious side-effects. Interferon and transfer factor have also been tried but have not proved to have an established place in therapy.

Neuromyelitis optica (Devic's disease)

Neuromyelitis optica is probably a specific form of multiple sclerosis. It is characterized by the rapid onset of bilateral optic neuritis and transverse myelitis separated by days or weeks. Either the spinal or optic nerve lesion may appear first.

Diffuse cerebral sclerosis

This is a condition first described by Schilder in which there is massive demyelination of the cerebral white matter characterized clinically by progressive visual failure, spasticity and dementia. It is very rare and it probably represents a heterogeneous group of disorders.

Acute disseminated encephalomyelitis

Acute disseminated encephalomyelitis is acute demyelination of the white matter of the brain and spinal cord, characterized pathologically by perivascular cellular infiltration and perivenous demyelination. It usually follows exanthematous viral infections such as measles, chicken pox, rubella and smallpox (postinfectious encephalomyelitis), but may also follow vaccinations (postvaccinial encephalomyelitis).

The onset is commonly about 5–20 days after the exanthem or vaccination and the condition has an immune basis. The onset is usually abrupt with headache, drowsiness, fever and sometimes convulsions. There is a combination of pyramidal tract, cerebellar and brainstem signs. The mortality rate may be as high as 30%; in the remainder of cases, recovery occurs with a variable degree of neurological deficit.

References

Hallpike J.F., Adams C.W. and Tourtelotte W.W. (eds) (1983) *Multiple Sclerosis*. Chapman and Hall, London.

McDonald W.I. and Silberberg D.H. (eds) (1986) *Multiple Sclerosis*. Butterworths, London.

Matthews W.B., Acheson E.D., Batchelor J.R. and Weller R.O. (eds) (1985) *McAlpine's Multiple Sclerosis*. Churchill-Livingstone, Edinburgh.

Poser C.M., Paty D.W. Scheinberg L., McDonald, W.I. and Ebers G.C. (eds) (1984) *The Diagnosis of Multiple Sclerosis*. Thieme-Stratton, New York.

21 Degenerative Diseases

Dementia

Intellectual deterioration may be caused by cerebrovascular disease (multi-infarct dementia), head injury, encephalitis (such as Creutzfeldt-Jakob disease and subacute sclerosing panencephalitis), or any other cause of multifocal or diffuse cortical disease. Primary degenerative brain disease develops in a number of conditions including Alzheimer's and Pick's disease (Chapter 14), Huntington's disease and Parkinson's disease (Chapter 11), and in familial myoclonic epilepsy and some other multisystem degenerations. The subject of dementia is considered separately in Chapter 14.

Motor system diseases

Motor neurone disease (amyotrophic lateral sclerosis)
(pp. 105–6)

This is a degenerative disorder of upper and lower motor neurones that presents most commonly in later life. In about 10–20% of cases there is autosomal dominant inheritance. Progressive weakness leads to death in a mean of about 4 years from the time of diagnosis. There are characteristic pathological changes of degeneration in the anterior horn cells of the spinal cord, the motor nuclei of the medulla and the corticospinal tracts (Fig. 8.7).

The presenting clinical features are variable depending upon the extent of involvement of lower and upper motor neurones and may consist predominantly of muscle wasting or spasticity, or a combination of the two. There are three recognized modes of presentation:

Progressive muscular atrophy Muscular wasting and fasciculation are usually noticed first in the small muscles of the hand or in the lower limbs, accompanied by foot-drop, and spread slowly to involve all muscles except those concerned with eye movements. Painful muscle cramps are a common complaint.

Progressive lateral sclerosis   This is a rare variant in which signs of upper motor neurone degeneration, spasticity and hyper-reflexia, precede those of lower motor neurone involvement. Most commonly upper and lower motor neurone signs occur together giving a characteristic combination of wasted muscles with increased reflexes in the affected limbs (*amyotrophic lateral sclerosis*).

Progressive bulbar palsy

Impairment of bulbar function (swallowing, coughing and articulation of speech) may be the initial disability, but always develops at some stage of the disease with atrophy and fasciculation of the tongue. The upper motor neurone (corticobulbar tract) is often involved as well so that voluntary elevation of the palate is less than that provoked by the gag reflex, and the jaw jerk is increased (pseudobulbar palsy). Pseudobulbar palsy is also characterized by loss of control over emotional reactions so that patients may laugh and cry inappropriately. Dysphagia may be aggravated by spasm of the cricopharyngeus muscle and partially relieved by its division (myotomy).

The cause is unknown and there is no specific treatment. The management involves helping patients cope with various symptoms as they arise and providing assistance in the home when they become disabled. Many patients derive comfort from membership of the Amyotrophic Lateral Sclerosis (ALS) Society. Death is usually caused by bulbar and respiratory weakness with inhalational pneumonia. By mutual agreement between patient, relatives and medical staff, resuscitation measures are usually avoided in the terminal phase when relief of pain and distress becomes more important than the prolongation of life.

Chronic proximal spinal muscular atrophy (Kugelberg-Welander syndrome)

This is a mild, slowly progressive disorder with benign prognosis; it is compatible with a normal life-span. Inheritance is usually autosomal recessive, but dominant and X-linked forms have also been described. The onset is in childhood or adolescence with difficulty in walking because of hip-girdle weakness. Proximal muscles in upper and lower limbs are mainly affected and the distribution of muscle weakness may cause the condition to be mistaken for muscular dystrophy. However fasciculations are often seen and the neurogenic nature of the disorder is confirmed by EMG and muscle biopsy. Bulbar musculature is spared and upper motor neurone signs are rarely present. There is no specific therapy.

Acute infantile spinal muscular atrophy (Werdnig-Hoffman disease)

This is a rapidly progressive anterior horn cell degeneration with an autosomal recessive inheritance. It may be apparent at birth (floppy baby syndrome) or develop during the first 6 months of life. The mean survival is 6 months and most children are dead by 18 months of age. A more slowly progressive variant is recognized.

Hereditary spastic paraplegia

The pure form of hereditary spastic paraplegia is a degeneration of the corticospinal pathways, usually inherited as an autosomal dominant characteristic, causing progressive spasticity with hyper-reflexia and extensor plantar responses. The legs are primarily affected and the arms are rarely involved. The age of onset and degree of disability vary in different families.

There are complicated forms of hereditary spastic paraplegia in which the features of spasticity may be combined with muscle wasting (amyotrophy), mental retardation, ataxia, optic atrophy, extrapyramidal features or sensory neuropathy.

Extrapyramidal disease

Parkinson's disease, Huntington's disease, dystonia musculorum deformans and Wilson's disease are described in Chapter 11.

A mixed pyramidal and extrapyramidal degeneration of late onset, characterized by impairment of voluntary vertical eye movements, axial rigidity and gait disturbance, is known as progressive supranuclear palsy (Steele-Richardson syndrome).

A rare autosomal recessive disorder is associated with deposition of iron in the basal ganglia (Hallevorden-Spatz disease). It runs a slowly progressive course over 10–20 years with extrapyramidal and pyramidal features.

Hereditary ataxias

The hereditary ataxias are a group of disorders which are classified according to their clinical, genetic and pathological features.

Friedreich's ataxia

This is a disease with an autosomal recessive inheritance with onset under the age of 25 years (mean 12 years), the first symptom usually being ataxia of gait. Other clinical features are dysarthria, incoordination, absent reflexes in the lower limbs, impaired position and vibration sense, extensor plantar responses, pes cavus, scoliosis and cardiomyopathy. Diabetes may be a complication. Pathologically it is characterized by degeneration of the spinocerebellar tracts, posterior columns, corticospinal tracts, and of the cell bodies in the dorsal root ganglia with their large afferent fibres mediating proprioception and tendon reflexes (Fig. 8.7). Optic atrophy and deafness may also be associated. The condition is progressive and the mean age of death is 37 years, usually due to heart failure, pneumonia or diabetes. Treatment is limited to supportive measures and the management of cardiac dysrhythmias or failure and diabetes in some patients. Friedreich's Ataxia Associations and other support groups exist in most large cities.

Other early onset cerebellar ataxias

In some types of early onset cerebellar ataxia the tendon jerks are retained (in contrast to Friedreich's ataxia) and scoliosis, impaired proprioception, cardiac abnormalities, and diabetes are less common than in Friedreich's ataxia.

Another form of cerebellar ataxia in which the pathological changes are those of cerebello-olivary atrophy was first described by Holmes. Since the degenerative changes are confined to the cerebellum and its connections and to the spinal cord, and peripheral nerves are normal, there are no associated pyramidal tract or peripheral nerve signs and the reflexes remain intact. Inheritance is usually autosomal recessive.

Progressive cerebellar ataxia of early onset may be associated with myoclonus. This autosomal recessive disorder is known as the Ramsay-Hunt syndrome. The age of onset is usually between the ages of 5 and 15 years. This syndrome, and related system degenerations with myoclonus, are prevalent in countries surrounding the Baltic Sea and are included in the term 'Baltic myoclonus'. Myoclonus may also be associated with cerebellar degeneration in storage diseases (Lafora body disease, cerebral lipidosis), and mitochondrial myopathy.

Late onset cerebellar ataxia

Olivopontocerebellar atrophy is a form of progressive cerebellar ataxia of middle life which usually has an autosomal dominant mode of inheritance. Pontine and midbrain structures degenerate in addition to the cerebellum, and clinical features include ataxia, dysarthria, nystagmus, pyramidal tract signs, optic atrophy and ophthalmoplegia.

Other forms of late onset cerebellar ataxia exist in which there is no family history.

Optic atrophy

Optic atrophy may be found in combination with many of the disorders described above.

Leber's optic atrophy is an hereditary disorder in its own right, affecting predominantly males, but the pattern of inheritance is not clear. Central vision deteriorates, often suddenly, in the second or third decades of life.

Retinitis pigmentosa is also more common in males and may be of recessive or dominant inheritance. It starts with night blindness, followed by peripheral constriction of the visual fields. A network of pigment can be seen extending throughout the retina, sparing the macula. It may be associated with other hereditary disorders such as hereditary ataxias, familial spastic paraplegia, ocular myopathy, polyneuropathy and deafness (Refsum's disease), and a syndrome of obesity, hypogonadism, mental retardation, and syndactyly (Laurence-Moon-Biedl syndrome).

Deafness

Hereditary perceptive (nerve) deafness may be associated with many neurological disorders, such as optic atrophy, polyneuropathy, familial myoclonic epilepsy and hereditary ataxias.

Peripheral neuropathy (see Chapter 5)

Peroneal muscular atrophy (Charcot-Marie-Tooth Disease)

This is a predominantly motor neuropathy, usually with autosomal dominant inheritance. It has been separated on histological grounds into hereditary sensorimotor neuropathy (HMSN) type I with demyelination and hypertrophic changes and HMSN type II with axonal degeneration. Another form of Charcot-Marie-Tooth disease is known as the Roussy-Lévy syndrome, and is associated with tremor.

Hypertrophic polyneuropathy (Dejerine-Sottas disease HMSN III)

This is a recessively inherited demyelinating neuropathy with hypertrophic changes that becomes clinically apparent in the first decade. Sensory disability is greater and the condition progresses more rapidly than Charcot-Marie-Tooth disease.

Hereditary sensory neuropathy

This is a dominantly inherited neuropathy in which sensory symptoms and signs are predominant, although some members of affected families may develop distal wasting resembling that of Charcot-Marie-Tooth disease. Lightning (stabbing) pains may be a distressing symptom. Loss of pain sensation may be so profound that joints are destroyed (Charcot joints), and trophic ulcers develop on the feet for want of protective reflexes.

Congenital insensitivity to pain

These are rare syndromes of universal analgesia; pain pathways may be abnormal in either the peripheral or the central nervous system. Congenital indifference to pain is a condition in which pain can be perceived but is disregarded.

Rare metabolic neuropathies

Refsum's disease is an autosomal recessive polyneuropathy associated with cerebellar ataxia, retinitis pigmentosa and nerve deafness, and an increase in blood phytanic acid. Other metabolic neuropathies are caused by disorders of lipoprotein metabolism (a-beta-lipoproteinaemia, or Bassen-Kornzweig syndrome, associated with acanthocytosis; an-alpha-lipopoteinaemia, or Tangier disease), by accumulation of sulfatide (metachromatic leucodystrophy) or of amyloid (familial amyloid neuropathy).

Familial dysautonomia

This is a rare congenital, recessively inherited polyneuropathy with defective autonomic function (Riley-Day syndrome).

Muscular dystrophy (see Chapter 6)

Neurocutaneous syndromes (the phakomatoses)

Tuberous sclerosis

This is a congenital disorder, occurring sporadically or as an autosomal dominant condition, characterized by areas of ectodermal or mesodermal hyperplasia in the skin, nervous and other systems. The abnormal gene has been assigned to the long arm of chromosome 9. It usually presents as epilepsy in a child with some degree of mental retardation and is recognized initially by the nature of the skin lesions. The following anomalies may be present.

Skin Reddish papules over the nasolabial folds, cheek and chin ('adenoma sebaceum'). Fibrotic areas in the skin, usually on the back, known as shagreen (sharkskin) patches. Leaf-shaped areas of hypopigmentation on the trunk or limbs — 'ash leaf patches'. Tumours of the nail-bed (subungual fibromas).

Nervous system Tubers of astrocytes and giant cells are scattered throughout the brain and in the walls of the lateral ventricles and are the cause of epilepsy in this condition. They commonly calcify and may be seen readily on a CT scan and sometimes on a plain radiograph of the skull.

Retina Gliomatous nodules (phakomas) may be seen in the vicinity of the optic disc.

Other organs Rhabdomyomas of the heart, lung cysts ('honeycomb lungs'), and benign tumours or cysts of the kidney, liver and other organs are not uncommon.

Neurofibromatosis

There are two forms of this disorder. The first is associated with bilateral acoustic neuromas and sometimes neuromas on other cranial or spinal nerves. Skin lesions may not be conspicuous. This variety is now called 'acoustic neurofibromatosis'. The second form has a more benign outlook and the term 'Von Recklinghausen's disease' is now restricted to this variety. Inheritance is autosomal dominant. The following manifestations of neurofibromatosis may be present in any one patient.

Skin Areas of skin the colour of milk coffee (*café au lait* patches) are found of larger size and in greater number than in the general population. Some 80% of patients have six or more large patches. Multiple freckles may be seen in the axilla or over the lower abdomen, buttocks and upper thighs. Spots of depigmentation may be found in the skin elsewhere.

Cutaneous tumours may feel hard or soft to palpation. Firm subcutaneous nodules may be felt attached to nerves and overgrowth of subcutaneous fibrous tissue may produce deformities.

Iris A small hamartoma may be seen as a pale spot in the iris in most instances.

Peripheral nerves Peripheral nerves may be palpable in the posterior triangle of the neck, elbow or popliteal fossa. Nerve palsies may develop as a 'mononeuritis multiplex'.

Brain Neuromas on the acoustic, trigeminal or other cranial nerves. Gliomas and meningiomas are also more common in this condition.

Spinal cord Tumours of spinal nerves may compress the spinal cord, enlarge the appropriate intervertebral foramen and form a paravertebral mass ('button-hole neurofibromas'). Spinal root or cauda equina tumours may simulate root compression by a cervical or lumbar disc lesion but radicular pain is usually the first and most persistent symptom of radicular neurofibromas.

Other organs A phaeochromocytoma develops in about 0.5% of patients with neurofibromatosis. From the other aspect, neurofibromatosis is present in 5–20% of patients with phaeochromocytoma.

Sturge-Weber syndrome

In this condition, there is an association of a capillary haemangioma (port-wine stain) in the distribution of the first division of the ophthalmic nerve with a meningeal naevus and calcification in the gyri of the underlying cortex. The calcification, which shows up as parallel lines in plain X-rays (tramline calcification), is readily seen in CT scans, and is usually more prominent over the posterior half of the affected hemisphere. The facial naevus may involve the eye, causing glaucoma. The intracranial anomaly is usually accompanied by a mild contralateral hemiparesis and focal (partial) motor seizures. The condition is not associated with intracerebral arteriovenous malformations, nor is there any tendency to subarachnoid haemorrhage. It is not usually familial.

Familial telangiectasia (Osler-Weber-Rendu disease)

Telangiecteses are seen as small red spots, blanching on pressure, on the skin and on the lips in this autosomal dominant disorder. Mucosal telangiecteses often give rise to epistaxis or intestinal bleeding. Telangiectasia is an uncommon cause of intracerebral or intraspinal haemorrhage but should be kept in mind when a young patient suffers a catastrophe of this sort without demonstrable cause.

Ataxia telangiectasia

This is an autosomal recessive disorder beginning with ataxia and choreoathetotic movements in the first decade of life, associated with telangiecteses on the conjunctiva and other areas of the face or neck. There is a deficiency of IgA and an immune deficiency state that renders the patient prone to repeated infection or the development of lymphoma. Death usually occurs in the second or third decade of life.

Von Hippel-Lindau disease

This association of retinal angioma with cerebellar haemangioblastoma may have autosomal dominant inheritance or may be sporadic. The tumour secretes erythropoietin which can cause polycythaemia. The lesions are treated independently by laser and surgical excision, respectively.

Storage diseases and other inherited metabolic abnormalities

Lysosomal storage diseases result from specific enzyme deficiencies that permit the accumulation of a metabolite that would normally be degraded. Some examples of cerebral lipidosis are given below.

Tay-Sachs disease

A disease of infancy, characterized by mental regression, pyramidal tract degeneration, myoclonus and the development of a cherry-red spot at the macula, ending in death by the age of 5 years. The deficient enzyme is hexosaminidase A and the accumulated metabolite is Gm_2 ganglioside. The condition is restricted to the Jewish race.

Juvenile cerebroretinal degeneration

Infantile, juvenile and adult forms of cerebral lipidosis are recognized in which macular degeneration, myoclonus, generalized seizures and mental retardation are salient features.

Metachromatic leukodystrophy

A sphingolipid storage disease caused by the absence of aryl sulfatase A, leading to the accumulation of sulfatide. There are infantile, juvenile and adult forms, with autosomal recessive inheritance. It is characterized by mental regression, pyramidal and cerebellar signs and peripheral neuropathy. The diagnosis may be confirmed by the presence of metachromatic granules in a nerve biopsy. The condition runs a progressively downhill course over a period of 5 years.

References

Adams R.D. and Victor M. (1985) *Principles of Neurology*, 3rd edn, Chapters 37, 39, 42. McGraw-Hill, New York.

Baraitser M. (1982) *The Genetics of Neurological Disorders*. Oxford University Press, Oxford.

Harding A.E. (1984) *The Hereditary Ataxias and Related Disorders*. Churchill Livingstone, London.

22 Headache

Pain pathways and headache mechanisms

Pain sensitive structures

Headache may arise from intracranial or extracranial structures and may be referred to the head from the eyes, sinuses or upper neck. The brain itself is insensitive to pain but the large intracranial arteries, veins, venous sinuses and parts of the dura may give rise to pain, referred to specific parts of the head. In general terms, structures in the anterior and middle cranial fossae refer pain to the anterior two-thirds of the head via the first division of the trigeminal nerve while pain from the posterior fossa is felt in the upper neck and occiput, being relayed by the second and third cervical roots. A dividing line between the anterior and posterior areas of referral may be drawn vertically above the ear. The external carotid artery and its frontal, temporal and middle meningeal branches also refer pain to the frontotemporal region via the first division of the trigeminal nerve. The occipital arteries and the joints of the upper cervical spine refer pain to the occiput through the C1–3 roots.

Referred pain

Pain referral is complicated by the fact that pain fibres from the head and face descend in the spinal tract of the trigeminal nerve to the upper three segments of the spinal cord where they synapse on the same second order neurones as afferent fibres from the C1–3 roots (Fig. 22.1). This means that pain originating from the upper cervical spine can be referred to the eye and forehead of the same side and that fronto-orbital headache may extend backwards like a bar of pain to the upper neck.

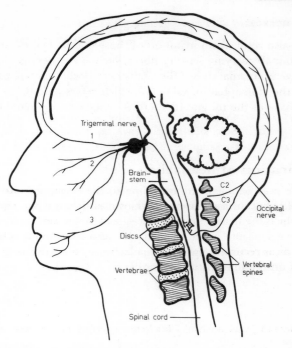

Fig. 22.1 Pain pathways from the head. The spinal tract of the trigeminal nerve descends to the upper three segments of the cervical cord where it synapses on second order neurones that also receive afferents from the second and third cervical roots. This convergence permits referral of pain from the head to neck and vice versa. (From Lance, 1975, with permission of Charles Scribner's Sons, New York.)

The upper cervical cord can therefore be regarded as a centre for the transmission of head and neck pain.

Endogenous pain control system

Pain transmission in the cord is controlled by tracts descending from the brainstem, a serotoninergic pathway from nucleus raphe magnus of the medulla and a noradrenergic pathway from the region of the locus coeruleus, which act on the first order synapse indirectly through interneurones that employ enkephalins or GABA as a transmitter (Fig. 4.4). Failure of the endogenous pain control system could permit spontaneous aching to be felt in the head, neck or both sides. Depletion of monoamine transmitters in this system may be a factor in essential or idiopathic headaches such as tension headache and migraine.

Cranial nerves

Pain can also result from irritation of those cranial nerves (other than the trigeminal) carrying sensory fibres, such as the nervus intermedius of the seventh cranial nerve; the vagus nerve, which refers pain to the ear, and the glossopharyngeal nerve which refers pain to the pharynx and the base of the tongue (deep to the angle of the mandible).

Classification of headache

Headache may be classified according to the presumed site of origin (Table 22.1) but the most useful working classification is to consider the way in which the headache presents — as a single severe episode, as a progressive subacute onset of headache, as a continuous ache of long standing or as recurrent episodic headaches — since this helps to focus the mind on the differential diagnosis.

Table 22.1   Classification of headaches according to presumed site of origin

---

Cranium
1. Expanding lesions within the cranial bones stretching the periosteum.
2. Inflammation of cranium or scalp.

Extracranial arteries
1. Temporal arteritis.

Cranial nerves
1. Excessive stimulation of trigeminal or glossopharyngeal nerves (e.g. headache on eating ice-cream, diving into cold water).
2. Distortion or inflammation of cranial nerves.
   Tumour, aneurysm.
   Tolosa-Hunt syndrome (a recurrent granulomatous disorder affecting the region of the superior orbital fissure). Raeder's paratrigeminal neuralgia (lesions involving the pericarotid sympathetic plexus, thus producing a partial Horner's syndrome, as well as the first division of the trigeminal nerve).
   Gradenigo's syndrome (lesions of the apex of the temporal bone involving the first division of the trigeminal and the sixth cranial nerve).
   Postherpetic neuralgia.
3. Trigeminal and glossopharyngeal neuralgia.
4. Atypical facial pain.

Table 22.1 (*continued*)

Referred pain
1. From eyes, ear, nose and throat, teeth, and neck.

Intracranial sources of headache
1. Vasodilatation caused by one of the following:
   (a) concussion
   (b) an epileptic fit (postictal)
   (c) pressor reactions
       (i) phaeochromocytoma
       (ii) tyramine ingestion by a patient taking monoamine oxidase inhibitors
       (iii) sexual excitement at orgasm
       (iv) malignant hypertension
   (d) toxic effects
       (i) systemic infections or intoxications
       (ii) 'hangover' headache after alcohol intoxication
       (iii) foreign protein reactions
       (iv) withdrawal of caffeine after excessive intake
       (v) some medications such as indomethacin
   (e) metabolic disturbances
       (i) hypoxia
       (ii) hypoglycaemia
       (iii) hypercapnia
   (f) vasodilator agents
2. Meningeal irritation
   (a) Subarachnoid haemorrhage
   (b) Meningitis, encephalitis
3. Displacement of intracranial vessels
   (a) Space-occupying lesions — tumour, haematoma, abscess
   (b) Increased intracranial pressure — obstructive hydrocephalus, cerebral oedema, benign intracranial hypertension
   (c) Reduced intracranial pressure — post-lumbar puncture headache
4. Exertional and cough headache of benign aetiology

Episodic headaches of uncertain mechanism
1. Migraine
2. Cluster headache
3. Acute cerebral vascular insufficiency

Tension headache
1. Primary muscle overcontraction
2. Secondary to other factors such as eye strain, temporomandibular joint dysfunction (Costen's syndrome), cervical spondylosis
3. Idiopathic chronic tension headaches
4. Tension-vascular headache

Psychogenic headache
1. Secondary to a delusional, conversion or hypochondriacal state

Acute severe headache

When a patient suddenly complains of severe headache for the first time, the presence or absence of fever and neck rigidity is of the greatest importance, since some of the more serious causes [such as (a) and (c) below] are associated with the signs of meningeal irritation.

(a) Subarachnoid haemorrhage;

(b) cerebral haemorrhage or infarction;

(c) encephalitis or meningitis;

(d) systemic infections, such as influenza or the exanthemata;

(e) acute obstruction of CSF pathways;

(f) sudden gross elevation of blood pressure, such as in acute nephritis, malignant hypertension or other causes of hypertensive crisis;

(g) sinusitis, usually with tenderness over the frontal or maxillary sinuses. Sphenoidal and ethmoidal sinusitis cause a mid-frontal headache;

(h) ocular disturbances, such as acute angle-closure glaucoma;

(i) injury to the head or upper neck;

(j) the first episode of migraine or other conditions considered later as *recurrent episodic headaches*.

Progressive subacute headache

This is a *sinister pattern of headache*, when the patient experiences a headache which may fluctuate in intensity but progressively becomes more severe over a period of days, weeks or months. If the headache is made worse by coughing, sneezing or straining, it suggests an intracranial origin with dilatation or displacement of intracranial vessels or obstruction of the ventricular system. If the headache is associated with drowsiness, mental changes, epileptic fits or any form of neurological deficit, the probability of an intracranial space-occupying lesion or chronic meningitis becomes greater. In the older age group, the possibility of temporal arteritis must always be considered. The progressive subacute headache always requires investigation. Possible causes include the following.

Space-occupying lesions: subdural haematoma, intracranial tumour and cerebral abscess

Infections of the ear may spread to the apex of the petrous temporal bone, causing pain in the first division of the trigeminal nerve and paralysis of the sixth cranial nerve (Gradenigo's syndrome). They may also cause thrombosis of the lateral venous sinus with resulting increase in the intracranial pressure (otitic hydrocephalus) or may form abscesses in the temporal lobe or cerebellum. Infections of the frontal sinus may cause an extradural or a cerebral abscess in the frontal lobe. Cerebral abscesses may also be embolic from infection in the lung or heart (acute or subacute bacterial endocarditis), or be caused by septi-caemia.

Chronic meningitis

(a) Tuberculous or cryptococcal (torula) meningitis.
(b) Syphilis.
(c) Meningitis carcinomatosa. Diffuse infiltration of the meninges by some tumours, such as primary lymphoma and secondary melanoma, which may simulate meningitis both in clinical presentation and in lowering CSF glucose levels below 2 μmol/l in the manner of a bacterial infection.

Benign intracranial hypertension (BIH)

If a patient presents with progressive headache and papilloedema, and elevated CSF pressure, and a space-occupying lesion or infectious process has been excluded, the diagnosis of BIH must be considered (see Chapter 18, p. 259).

Temporal arteritis

Temporal arteritis affects women more than men in the ratio 3:1, mostly over the age of 50 years although one patient aged 35 years has been reported. The condition may affect intracranial arteries, particularly the ophthalmic artery, as well as extracranial arteries and occasionally branches of the aorta (coronary, renal and iliac arteries). In about half the cases it is associated with diffuse aching in muscles and joints (poly-myalgia rheumatica). The condition is probably an immune disorder and the characteristic pathological change is thickening of the intima, fibrosis and cellular infiltration of the media with giant-cell formation and thrombus formation in the lumen.

In classical cases, the extracranial arteries are palpable and tender but the condition should be suspected in any elderly patient with pro-gressive headache, particularly if associated with generalized body aching and malaise. One pathognomonic symptom is claudication of the jaw muscles — aching of the jaw on repeated chewing caused by involve-ment of the branches of the external carotid artery.

The ESR is elevated above 40 mm/h in two-thirds of patients but note that a normal ESR does not exclude the condition. If the index of suspicion is high, one temporal artery should be biopsied since it is important to make the diagnosis with certainty. Corticosteroid therapy can be started before temporal artery biopsy and may have to be continued for months and possibly years. The importance of early diagnosis is that the ophthalmic artery becomes involved in 20–50% of cases in various reported series and causes rapid loss of vision in the affected eye. The chance of this complication is reduced to half by the use of steroids.

Chronic continuous headache

A constant headache, present most of the time for most days of the week over a long period of time is unlikely to be caused by any structural abnormality and is a form of *essential headache* which is closely linked with the emotional state of the patient. The following forms of chronic continuous headache may be encountered.

Tension headache

This is a tight, pressing or band-like sensation felt on top of or around the head, and is usually bilateral. It affects women about twice as often as men and may start at any age. Fifteen per cent of patients recall their headaches starting under the age of 10 years.

Tension headache used to be considered to be the result of constant overcontraction of the frontal, temporal and occipital muscles and there is little doubt that this plays an important part in some patients who are able to overcome their symptoms by learning to relax the appropriate muscles. Careful controlled observations have now shown that there is no statistical difference in the degree of muscle contraction between most sufferers of tension headache and normal controls and, moreover, there is no difference in pain threshold between the two groups. Some authors have considered tension headache to be one end of a spectrum which embraces 'tension-vascular' headache, common migraine and classical migraine and have postulated that a defect in monoamine neurotransmitters and in the endogenous pain control system are common factors in all essential headaches.

Although the basic cause is unknown, treatment is directed at the following factors.

Physical abnormalities   (a) Imbalance of the bite. Some patients have an uneven bite which throws strain on one temporomandibular joint, with the development of a clicking noise in the joint and pain radiating over the face and head from the affected joint (Costen's syndrome). Dental attention is required to correct the bite, but equally important is the reduction of excessive jaw clenching (bruxism) and the underlying anxiety state which is often present.

(b) Cervical spondylosis. Spasm of cervical muscles may be secondary to degenerative changes in the cervical spine and may respond to manipulative or other therapy for the neck problem.

(c) Eye strain. Ocular imbalance or refractive errors may be a source of tension and should be corrected. The subject should sit in a comfortable chair at work or school, adjusted to the height appropriate for the desk to ensure good posture, with lighting adjusted to the correct angle for comfort.

Psychological factors   In some patients exacerbations of headache may clearly be linked with sources of stress and may be helped by psychological counselling, alteration of life-style or readjustment of stresses. In other patients problems may be either inapparent or insoluble.

Other forms of treatment consist of muscle relaxation or pharmacotherapy. A course of relaxation training may be highly beneficial in a well-motivated patient. Various forms of biofeedback may assist relaxation but do not substantially improve the result. Courses of relaxation training are now conducted by many hospitals, community health centres and physiotherapists or psychologists.

Pharmacotherapy involves the use of tricyclic antidepressants, particularly amitriptyline, which are particularly helpful in those who tolerate them well. It is advisable to start with one half of a 25 mg tablet of amitriptyline at night then gradually increase to 3 tablets (75 mg) as a single nocturnal dose if there are no untoward side-effects such as drowsiness or confusion. Improvement is usually noted within a week and the treatment can be continued for 6 months before slowly weaning off medication to see whether improvement can be maintained by relaxation alone. Tranquillizers such as the benzodiazepines may also be used if necessary.

Tension-vascular headache

This term is applied to chronic daily tension headache with superimposed exacerbations of more severe pain, unilateral or bilateral, which resembles that of a mild migraine headache. This is treated along the same lines as tension headache but propranolol and pizotifen may be useful medication as described for migraine. Methysergide is not usually effective in tension-vascular headache.

Atypical facial pain

A constant pain, usually described as tight or boring, localized to one area of the lower face, particularly the nasolabial angle but may spread across the cheeks, bridge of the nose or other areas. It may come on after minor trauma such as dental extraction and persist indefinitely, defying all surgical measures including section of the trigeminal nerve. The aetiology is unknown. Management is along the same lines as for tension headache. The combination of amitriptyline and thioridazine (Melleril) will usually reduce the intensity of the pain and, in the present state of knowledge, the patient has to learn to live with the residual discomfort.

Postherpetic neuralgia

This complication of herpes zoster is more common as age advances. Once it has developed, it is intractable but may be suppressed by the combination recommended above for atypical facial pain.

Post-traumatic headache

There are many varieties of post-traumatic headache, often complicated by the anxiety (and sometimes desire for financial gain) engendered by legal proceedings which are often protracted for many years. The following syndromes are recognized:

Postconcussional headache   which affects only about 40% of patients and clears up rapidly.

Post-traumatic migraine   which may be limited to the vascular distribution of the area of scalp injured and is managed along the same lines as migraine.

Episodic unilateral headaches   resembling cluster headache following a blow to the carotid artery ('dysautonomic cephalgia'). This is very rare and is said to respond to propranolol.

Whiplash syndrome   This is an 'upper cervical syndrome' from disruption of soft tissues and zygapophysial joints in the upper cervical spine caused by a rapid acceleration of the body with passive extension of the neck, for example when the patient is sitting in a car hit from the rear. Pain is referred to the occiput. Treatment includes the application of heat, wearing of a surgical collar and the injection of a local anaesthetic agent and hydrocortisone into tender areas.

Tension headache   is often seen in conjunction with the other varieties.

Recurrent episodic headaches

These have been called *vascular headaches* in the past because scalp arteries and veins dilate in some patients and the pain may be throbbing in character and relieved by pressure over the appropriate vessels. This may be too simplistic a view as there are many other factors involved.

Migraine

Migraine is the most common of the episodic headaches and affects some 10% of males and 20% of females at some time of their lives. Some 25% of sufferers date the onset of their attacks from childhood, the incidence progressively increasing and remaining equal in both sexes until puberty, after which age women are affected twice as often as men.

Migraine is termed *classical* if the headache is preceded by neurological symptoms such as blurred vision, flashes of light, jittering zig-zags of light (*fortification spectra*) or, less commonly, paraesthesiae and dysphasia. These persist for 10–60 min and then commonly fade away as the headache starts although they may continue into the headache phase. There may be vague premonitory symptoms of elation ('feeling on top of the world'), hunger, thirst or drowsiness for up to 24 h before the migraine attack.

If the headache appears without any prodromal symptoms, it is known as *common migraine*. If the neurological symptoms develop and subside slowly without a headache ensuing, they are called *migraine equivalents*.

Variations on the theme of migraine include:

Vertebrobasilar migraine   The association of visual, brainstem and cerebellar disturbances, often leading to syncope, preceding or accompanied by headache. It is attributed to vasospasm in the vertebrobasilar circulation and resembles a slow-motion episode of the vertebrobasilar insufficiency encountered as a form of cerebral vascular disease.

Retinal migraine   A rare disorder in which loss of vision is limited to one eye as a result of retinal ischaemia, rather than to one or both homonymous visual fields as commonly encountered with the occipital lobe ischaemia of classical migraine.

Ophthalmoplegic migraine   A transient Horner's syndrome or, conversely, dilatation of one pupil, is not uncommon during a severe migraine attack. The term *ophthalmoplegic migraine* is reserved for the appearance of paralysis of one or more of the cranial nerves supplying the extraocular muscles, usually the third nerve, at the height of migraine headache. It is probably a transient ischaemic neuropathy, which may persist after repeated episodes.

Facial migraine   Recurrent episodes resembling migraine in which pain affects the eye, cheek and chin rather than the head.

Hemiplegic migraine   Hemiplegia may develop before or during a migraine headache. This form usually affects families as a dominant characteristic.

Complicated migraine   Neurological deficit persisting more than 24 h after the end of migraine headache. A permanent deficit may result from vascular thrombosis, particularly in young women taking a contraceptive pill.

Characteristics of migraine headache
Migraine is characteristically episodic, separated by intervals of freedom. It is unilateral in two-thirds of patients, commonly affecting the frontotemporal region, radiating to the occiput. The headache is usually accompanied by nausea (90%), vomiting (60%) or diarrhoea (20%). Most patients (80%) become sensitive to light and most are acutely aware of noise and smells during the headache. Fluid retention is common at the onset of headache and polyuria is noticed as the headache subsides. The scalp becomes tender on the affected side in two-thirds of patients.

The migraine personality
Migrainous patients are not more intelligent than their peers or more subject to stress but react more strongly to stress. There is a family history of migraine in about 50% of patients.

Precipitating factors
Intrinsic   Many patients with migraine have attacks with a regularity that suggests that the episodes are being triggered by some internal biological clock. Such rhythms may be: monthly, linked with the menstrual cycle (the trigger for menstrual migraine is probably the drop in

oestradiol level); weekly, associated with weekends or a particular week-day; nightly, awakening the patient in the phase of rapid eye movement (REM) sleep.

These internal rhythms may be altered by metabolic factors such as hypoglycaemia or by external triggers.

Extrinsic   Some patients state that their attacks are brought on by: (i) excessive afferent stimulation, such as flickering light, loud noise, strong perfumes or compression of scalp nerves (e.g. 'swim-goggle migraine'); (ii) a sharp blow to the head, such as 'heading the ball' in soccer ('footballer's migraine'); (iii) certain rich foods such as chocolates and other fatty foods. The specificity of food factors is dubious; (iv) stress or sudden relaxation after stress; (v) the ingestion of vasodilators such as alcohol, monosodium glutamate or drugs used in the management of angina pectoris and peripheral vascular disease. Physical exertion may have the same effect in producing vasodilatation and triggering a migraine headache.

Pathophysiology

Migraine is commonly associated with a diminution of cortical blood flow of about 20% which starts in the occipital region and slowly moves forward, accompanied by a spreading depression of cortical function. The headache phase may be accompanied by an increase in extracranial blood flow.

There is evidence that migraine attacks are associated with fluctuation in the levels of monoamines in the blood, possibly as a reflection of their neurotransmitter function within the central nervous system. Serotoninergic and noradrenergic pathways project from the brainstem to the cortical microcirculation as well as projecting to the spinal cord as part of the endogenous pain control system.

Blood serotonin and noradrenaline levels rise before the migraine attack and fall at the onset of the attack. It is postulated that hyperactivity followed by diminished activity in monaminergic transmission could produce the vascular changes of migraine and at the same time diminish inhibition of incoming afferent impulses, thus causing sensitivity to pain (and to light, sound and smell).

Platelet aggregation takes place in migraine, associated with release of serotonin from platelets, which may underlie the tendency to vascular thrombosis causing the neurological deficits of complicated migraine. The released serotonin, in combination with local formation of bradykinin and histamine, is thought to sensitize vessels to painful distension, thus adding a peripheral factor to the pain of migraine.

Management
Psychological counselling and relaxation therapy are employed as in the management of tension headache and may reduce the frequency of headache to half or less before any medication is used.

Treatment
Treatment of an acute attack consists of the following: (i) The administration of *ergotamine tartrate* orally, or by inhalation, rectal suppository or injection at the first sign of an attack aborts or diminishes the headache in 70% of patients. The usual oral dose of ergotamine tartrate is 1–2 mg, either alone (Lingraine) or combined with caffeine 100 mg (Cafergot), or with caffeine and an anti-emetic (e.g. Ergodryl). (ii) Naproxen is a possible alternative to ergotamine, 500 mg being taken at the onset and repeated in an hour if necessary. (c) Analgesics, best preceded by the injection or ingestion of metoclopramide (Maxolon) 10 mg to promote absorption and reduce nausea.

Prevention
Prevention of frequent attacks (two or more each month) by regular medication is known as 'interval therapy'. The following medications may be used.
(a) The beta-blocking agent propranolol (Inderal) 40 mg, starting with one-half tablet twice daily and increasing to two tablets three times daily if necessary and if it is tolerated well. It should not be used in asthmatics since it aggravates bronchospasm. Other side-effects include fatigue, postural hypotension and vivid dreams. Other beta-blockers effective in preventing migraine are those which have no intrinsic sympathomimetic activity, such as metoprolol, atenolol, and timolol.
(b) The antiserotonin, antihistamine agent pizotifen (Sandomigran) 0.5 mg. This is best given as a single nocturnal dose to avoid drowsiness, increasing slowly from one to six tablets at night until migraine is controlled or side-effects (drowsiness, increased appetite and weight gain) limit its use.
(c) The antiserotonin agent methysergide (Deseril). This may give rise to side-effects (indigestion, peripheral vasoconstriction, muscle aches) in one-third of patients if the full dose is started immediately. The patient should be advised to cut a tablet in half (an intricate procedure as the tablets are small and coated) and take one half tablet twice daily. The dose is then progressively increased to two tablets three times daily if necessary to control headache. Medication should be continued for 4 months, then discontinued for 1 month before starting again, to minimize the possibility of pleural or retroperitoneal fibrosis developing.

Such fibrotic side-effects are extremely rare (less than five per thousand) even when medication is continuous but patients should be advised to have a regular medical check-up and blood urea test every 3 months and to report if they experience chest or abdominal pains.

(d) Amitriptyline, which prevents re-uptake of serotonin, is also helpful in interval therapy of migraine.

(e) Non-steroidal anti-inflammatory drugs may also be useful.

(f) Calcium channel-blocking agents are being evaluated for their effectiveness in preventing migraine.

Cluster headache (migrainous neuralgia)

Cluster headache is an unusual unilateral headache syndrome (only 3% as common as migraine), affecting males in 85% of cases, which gains its name from the tendency to occur in bouts or clusters, lasting from weeks to months at a time, separated by months or years of freedom. During a bout, the patient is subject to brief attacks of severe pain, usually lasting 15 min to 2 h, which recur once or more in each 24-hour period, commonly at night.

The pain usually affects one eye and radiates upwards over the fronto-temporal region or downwards over the face. It is commonly associated with redness and watering of the eye and blockage of the nostril on the same side. In one-third or more of cases, a partial Horner's syndrome (ptosis and miosis) is noted on the affected side.

Treatment of episodic cluster headache consists of regular (interval) medication during the susceptible period.

(a) Ergotamine tartrate, given as 1–2 mg daily during the bout. It may be sufficient to give a nocturnal dose only if the attacks occur solely during the night. This is usually adequate to control the first or second bout.

(b) Methysergide, 1–2 mg three times daily, as for migraine, is used if ergotamine tartrate is ineffective.

(c) Prednisone, 75 mg daily, for 3 days, reducing rapidly to a dose just sufficient to prevent the attacks (usually about 25 mg daily), which is then maintained for the duration of the bout before weaning off slowly. This is effective in suppressing a bout in approximately 80% of cases.

In the acute episode, the inhalation of 100% oxygen stops the pain rapidly in most cases.

There are two variations on the theme of cluster headache. (i) Chronic cluster headache, in which pain recurs regularly without remission, in the manner of migraine. This form usually responds to medication with lithium carbonate, 250 mg two or three times daily, the dose being adjusted to provide a blood level of 0.7–1.0 mEq/l. Side-effects include tremor and confusion. (ii) Chronic paroxysmal hemi-crania, in which brief attacks of pain recur six or more times daily. This form is usually controlled rapidly by indomethacin, 25 mg three times daily.

Trigeminal neuralgia

Definition and pathophysiology   Trigeminal neuralgia is a degenerative condition of the trigeminal pathways, commonly caused by branches of the anterior or superior cerebellar arteries impinging on the root of the trigeminal nerve where it enters the pons, which causes severe stabbing pains in the distribution of one or more branches of the trigeminal nerve. Other causes include a small angioma or neuroma overlying the trigeminal root, or a plaque of multiple sclerosis at the root entry zone in the pons (which accounts for some 2–3% of cases of trigeminal neuralgia). Partial demyelination is thought to cause repetitive synchronous discharges of nerve fibres.

The condition is known as *tic douloureux* (a painful spasm) because of the lightning-like jabs of pain which are typical of the condition. It affects females more than males in the ratio 1.6 : 1 and usually starts after the age of 40 years, most commonly in the 50s. Most start in the second or third divisions, only 5% starting in the first division. Trigger factors include talking, chewing, swallowing, shaving, cleaning the teeth and wind blowing on the face. Trigger points are usually areas around the nose or lips which evoke a paroxysm if touched.

Episodic pattern   This pain may recur many times a day for weeks and months, and then may remit for months or years. This episodicity bears a superficial resemblance to cluster headache from which trigeminal neuralgia can be distinguished on every other ground (character and distribution of pain and lack of the features associated with cluster headache).

Examination   No abnormality is found on examination in idiopathic trigeminal neuralgia. If sensory loss is found, if the corneal response is depressed, if there is associated deafness on the side of pain, or if an aching pain persists between the characteristic stabs, some underlying lesion must be sought since acoustic and trigeminal neuromas and other posterior fossa tumours as well as intrinsic lesions such as multiple scle-rosis may be present with tic-like pains.

Management   The pain can usually be subdued by the use of carbamaze-pine (Tegretol), 200 mg three times daily, or phenytoin (Dilantin), 100 mg three times daily, or baclofen (Lioresal), 10–20 mg three times daily.

If the pain persists in spite of medical management, one of three surgical procedures can be undertaken.

(a) Posterior fossa exploration with separation of compressing arteries or veins from the trigeminal root. This is called the Jannetta procedure, but was first advocated by Dandy in 1932. It is appropriate for the younger patient as it preserves normal facial sensation.

(b) Thermocoagulation (radiofrequency lesion) of the Gasserian ganglion. This is relatively simple since the probe is inserted into the foramen ovale under local anaesthesia without the need for craniotomy. General anaesthesia is administered only during the process of coagulation which is otherwise very painful. This procedure is effective in most cases and preserves some sensation but troublesome dysaesthesiae develop in 2%.

(c) Intracranial section of the appropriate divisions of the trigeminal nerve.

Other episodic syndromes

Recurrent sinusitis This rarely presents any diagnostic difficulty in genuine cases. Most patients claiming to have episodic sinus headache suffer from migraine or one of its variants.

Paroxysmal hypertension Phaeochromocytoma may cause 'funny turns', accompanied by headache in 80% of cases. This is dealt with further in Chapter 17.

Transient ischaemic attacks of thrombo-embolic origin are associated with headache in about 25% of cases but the headache is usually overshadowed by the neurological symptoms.

Intermittent obstruction of CSF pathways This is more likely to present as a subacute progressive headache with fluctuations in intensity.

Recurrent meningitis This may be caused by a communication between CSF and nasopharynx or middle ear as a result of a fracture, most commonly through the cribriform plate. CSF rhinorrhoea may be observed as the patient bends forwards and the fluid can be distinguished from sinus secretions by the fact that it contains glucose. There is a recurrent aseptic meningitis known as Mollaret's meningitis which is probably a tendency to viral infections (? herpes simplex) in a patient with deficient immune mechanisms.

Recurrent subarachnoid haemorrhage from an angioma which, as a low pressure venous bleed, presents less hazard to life than haemorrhage from an aneurysm and may escape diagnosis on the first occasion, the bleed being labelled as 'viral meningo-encephalitis'. Beware of recurrent 'meningo-encephalitis'!

Benign syndromes such as headache during sexual intercourse, or on coughing or on exercise (benign only if an intracranial lesion has been excluded).

Investigation of headache

Patients with chronic continuous headache or episodic headaches usually require no more investigation than a careful history to establish the pattern of headache, followed by a physical examination of all systems.

Patients with an acute or subacute progressive pattern of headache usually require a CT scan of the brain as the initial investigation. Plain radiographs of the skull have little point if a CT scan is available but an X-ray of the chest should always be taken to exclude a carcinoma of the lung or other relevant condition. Bilateral carotid angiography may still be required even if the CT scan is negative since it may demonstrate bilaterally symmetrical subdural haematomas or an aneurysm which has escaped diagnosis by the other investigation.

A full blood count *and ESR* should always be obtained since temporal arteritis, collagen diseases, subacute bacterial endocarditis, multiple myeloma, leukaemia, anaemia and polycythaemia may all cause headache and may not be suspected on other grounds.

An electroencephalogram is rarely necessary if CT scanning and other diagnostic measures are available but can give valuable localizing information in cerebral abscess, herpes simplex encephalitis and some cases of cerebral tumour.

A lumbar puncture may be necessary to confirm the presence of encephalitis, meningitis, subarachnoid haemorrhage or benign intracranial hypertension. A CT scan of the brain is strongly advised to exclude a space-occupying lesion before lumbar puncture is attempted, since herniation of the brain through tentorium or foramen magnum can be caused by withdrawal of CSF from below, with serious and possibly fatal consequences.

If a headache history suggests one of the more sinister causes, immediate referral to a neurological unit is advisable.

References

Basbaum A.I. and Fields H.L. (1978) Endogenous pain control mechanisms: review and hypothesis. *Ann. Neurol.* **4**, 451–62.

Blau J.N. (ed.) (1987) *Migraine. Clinical and Research Aspects.* John Hopkins University Press, Baltimore.

Dalessio D.J. (1980) *Wolff's Headache and Other Head Pain,* 4th edn. Oxford University Press, New York.

Hopkins A. (ed.) (1988) *Headache. Problems in Diagnosis and Management.* W.B. Saunders, London.

Kudrow L. (1980) *Cluster Headache. Mechanisms and Management.* Oxford University Press, New York.

Lance J.W. (1982) *The Mechanism and Management of Headache,* 4th edn. Butterworths, London.

23 The Investigation and Treatment of Neurological Disorders

There is much more to treatment than the prescription of medication. Treatment starts from the moment patients recognize that you are taking their problem seriously and doing your best to find the cause. Sometimes a careful history and physical examination, followed by discussion and reassurance, will be all that is necessary. At all times the patient should be regarded as a partner in the therapeutic process.

The mental comfort of the patient

A medical examination can be an ordeal for some people. They may be afraid of giving silly answers to the doctor's questions, of taking off their clothes, of being prodded in sensitive and vulnerable areas and, when all is done, of being diagnosed as having some unpleasant or incurable disease. Tension is usually eased by a friendly approach and some words of explanation from the doctor as the examination progresses. Any discussion about the nature of the illness or advice about management must be expressed in words that the patient understands. Even intelligent and sophisticated patients may be vague about the location of their internal organs and what they do. Simple sketches may help your patient understand what is going on and what you propose to do about it.

The most important aspect of treatment is often the advice given to the patient — advice about personal relationships, life-style, family affairs, occupation, and personal habits such as diet, exercise, smoking, and the consumption of alcohol and drugs. Some conditions such as hyperventilation may be cured completely by explanation alone. Depression is common in neurological disorders, not only as an understandable reaction to disability but often as an integral part of the disorder. Antidepressant medication is then indicated and consultation with a psychiatrist is advisable for those with serious emotional disturbances.

Where should patients be treated? Are they able to continue work, should they rest at home or would they be better off in hospital? In any event, there should be close communication between general practitioner and specialist to ensure continuity of patient care.

Investigations

To what extent should the patient be investigated? A careful history and examination will reduce and may eliminate the need for any invasive tests. If these are required, they should be planned sequentially in a rational manner. The patients should be informed about the reasons for any investigations, what exactly is to be done to them and then told the results as they come to hand. Where should the tests be done? Many procedures can now be done as an out-patient, saving the expense and stress of hospital admission.

Routine investigation

Should the patient be admitted to hospital, the only routine investigations need be a chest X-ray, blood count and ESR. Biochemical and other investigations should be ordered after logical consideration and not as a form-filling or computerized conditioned reflex.

Lumbar puncture

Except in an emergency, such as suspected acute meningitis, lumbar puncture is not usually carried out until a CT scan of the brain has excluded a space-occupying lesion. Lumbar puncture is done to examine the CSF pressure or constituents for certain specific indications and must never be regarded as 'routine' (see Chapter 18 on CSF). If a myelogram is to be performed to exclude compression of the spinal cord and roots, a CSF sample should be obtained at the same time. Serological tests for syphilis, human immune deficiency virus (HIV) or other infectious agents are ordered when appropriate on blood or CSF samples. At present, the patient's permission has to be obtained before HIV tests can be done.

Imaging techniques

Computerized axial tomography

A thin beam of X-rays scans the head or spine in a series of planes and the differential absorption of each area is calculated by computer and displayed as a pictorial representation of the structures scanned (Fig. 23.1)

Fig. 23.1 CT scan of brain. The dark low-density area in left hemisphere (arrowed) represents an infarct in the distribution of the middle cerebral artery.

CT scanning demonstrates hydrocephalus, cerebral atrophy and the majority of infarcts, haemorrhages, tumours and other intracranial lesions. An intravenous injection of contrast medium is given to display the vascular system and may demonstrate an aneurysm or arterio-venous malformation. Where the blood–brain barrier is defective, in the vicinity of tumours or infarcts for example, the contrast medium enters cerebral tissue and is seen as an area of enhancement on the scan. Some tumours and subdural haematomas in an isodense phase may escape detection. With modern CT scanners, useful pictures of the spinal cord and roots can be obtained to detect compressing lesions, especially if used in conjunction with myelography.

Magnetic resonance imaging (MRI)

MRI depends on a strong magnetic field orienting hydrogen ions in the body in a north–south direction, followed by the application of a lateral magnetic pulse to displace these ions. The field generated during this process and the return to the previous orientation is analysed by com-

Fig. 23.2 Magnetic resonance imaging (MRI) of brain. (a) Midline sagittal MRI scan showing the ventricular system and aqueduct with enlargement of the medulla by a glioma (arrowed). (b) Horizontal MRI scan of the same patient, demonstrating the medullary lesion (arrowed).

puter to depict anatomical structures as a function of their water content (Fig. 23.2). The technique is complementary to CT scan, is about three times more expensive, and has advantages in showing small lesions in the grey matter (hamartomas, 'cryptogenic' haemangiomas, and areas of gliosis producing epileptogenic foci), areas of demyelination, for example in multiple sclerosis (Fig. 23.3) and some infiltrating tumours such as pontine glioma that may elude the CT scan. MRI also gives beautiful pictures of the spinal column, cord and roots that may make a definitive diagnosis of spinal cord compression or intrinsic lesions such as syringomyelia.

Arteriography, angiography

Injection of a contrast medium into the circulation, usually by means of a catheter inserted into the femoral artery and insinuated into the appropriate artery, demonstrates the carotid or vertebrobasilar circulation. Aneurysms, angiomas and the blood supply to tumours can be demonstrated in this way. Smaller doses of the contrast agent can be used intra-arterially if the images are enhanced by computer (Digital Subtraction Angiography, DSA). The intravenous injection of large amounts of contrast medium will also demonstrate the arterial circulation by the DSA technique but is of less diagnostic value than intra-arterial injection.

Fig. 23.3 Magnetic resonance imaging of brain in multiple sclerosis. (a) White areas (arrowed) represent plaques in cerebral white matter. (b) Periventricular demyelination (arrows).

Isotope ventriculography

To determine the rate of clearance of CSF from the ventricular system, a radioactive isotope can be injected into the lumbar sac and the ventricular content of isotope monitored for 48 h thereafter. This technique is sometimes employed in the diagnosis of hydrocephalus and in the detection of leaks of CSF, e.g. CSF rhinorrhoea after head injuries.

Myelography

A water-soluble contrast medium is inserted into the CSF by lumbar puncture to outline the spinal cord and roots radiologically. Myelography is still the investigation of choice to determine the site and extent of spinal cord compression. It may be followed by CT scanning while the contrast medium is still present to provide more accurate information about structural change at certain segmental levels. The contrast medium may later enter the spinal cord and demonstrate a central lesion such as syringomyelia. It is important to discuss the patient's clinical signs with the radiologist so that the suspected level is thoroughly investigated. A lumbar myelogram is of no help in diagnosing a lesion of the thoracic cord! A CSF sample is usually taken for examination at the time of the insertion of the contrast medium. Sufficient fluid should be taken to allow for an electrophoretogram (EPG) of CSF proteins to determine whether an oligoclonal band is present in the globulin fraction.

Neurophysiological techniques

Electroencephalography

The electroencephalogram (EEG) is a recording by electrodes attached to the scalp of the electrical field generated by the neuronal activity of the underlying brain. Electrodes are distributed equidistantly over the scalp and the potential difference between two points is displayed on each channel of the EEG (bipolar recording). The field recorded from each electrode can also be compared with the mean of the potentials recorded from all scalp electrodes (average reference electrode) at that time, or with the mean of that from the immediately surrounding electrodes (source derivation). This is the closest one can get to monopolar recording since it is impossible to find a suitable site for an indifferent electrode in the body because of the all-pervasive ECG which registers in millivolts compared with the EEG in microvolts.

Normal EEG rhythms are designated alpha (8–13 Hz, originating from generators in the occipital region), beta (14–22 Hz, maximal over the sensorimotor area), theta (4–7 Hz, prominent in children and diminishing during adolescence, recorded mainly from the temporal regions) and delta (1–3 Hz, normal only in early childhood). Less common normal patterns are: the mu rhythm, of alpha frequency but shaped like the top of a picket fence or the Greek letter μ and distributed asymmetrically in the central regions; and lambda waves that are generated in the occipital region by saccadic eye movements when the eyes are open. The occipital alpha rhythm depends upon the synchronous discharge of cells in the visual cortex. It is attenuated when the eyes are open and cells are discharging asynchronously during visual processing.

The most common abnormal EEG patterns are listed below.

(a) Generalized slow activity, encountered in coma and any diffuse cerebral disorder.

(b) Localized slow activity, recorded over the site of any focal lesion such as an infarct, abscess, herpes simplex encephalitis, or tumour.

(c) Localized spike discharges or sharp waves, that indicate a potentially epileptogenic focus (Fig. 23.4).

(d) Generalized spike-wave discharges which are called typical if they are well-formed at 3 Hz and atypical if they are of higher or lower frequency or if their pattern includes multiple spikes (polyspike-wave complexes) (Fig. 23.5). Such patterns are commonly associated with epilepsy (see Chapter 16).

(e) Episodic discharges may recur regularly in certain pancortical disorders such as subacute sclerosing panencephalitis (SSPE), Creutzfeldt-Jakob disease, and metabolic encephalopathies.

1 s

Fig. 23.4 Electroencephalogram showing sharp-waves over an epileptogenic focus.

After recording the resting EEG, the patient is asked to hyperventilate for 2–3 min because the resulting hypocapnia induces vasoconstriction which brings out slow rhythms and may delineate a focal abnormality that previously escaped notice or may induce a paroxysm of spike-wave. At the conclusion of the record, the patient is exposed to a stroboscopic light flashing at varying frequencies to provoke seizure patterns in susceptible patients. Other techniques used to identify epileptic foci are *sleep recordings*, which may reveal abnormalities not evident when the subject is awake, and prolonged (6–8 h) *telemetric recordings*. There is considerable variation in the normal EEG and minor deviations can be erroneously designated as abnormal, or, even worse, as indicative of epilepsy or other cerebral disorders.

The EEG is essential for the accurate diagnosis of epilepsy and is of some assistance in determining the nature of some pancortical disturbances such as SSPE or Creutzfeldt-Jakob disease. It can confirm the clinical localization of some cerebral lesions but imaging techniques do this much more effectively. An EEG should never be requested without a clear idea of the question it is required to answer.

Cerebral evoked responses

The cerebral potential induced by an afferent volley in the visual, auditory or common sensory pathways is normally of much lower amplitude than the EEG rhythms and cannot be discerned amongst them. By aver-

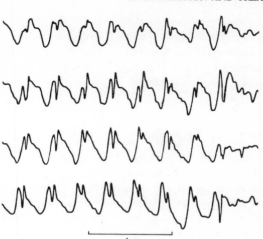

1 s

Fig. 23.5 Electroencephalogram showing typical 3 Hz spike and wave activity.

aging the EEG for a fixed time interval after the stimulus, the stimulus-related events become augmented while the random EEG rhythms are averaged out. The stimulus is usually a reversing black and white checker-board pattern or brief flash of light for the visual evoked response (VER), a click or pure tone for the brainstem auditory evoked response (BAER), and an electric shock applied to a peripheral nerve in the upper or lower limb for the somatosensory evoked response (SSER). The VER is used for the detection of past optic neuritis (see Chapters 9, 20; Fig. 20.2) and for monitoring visual pathways during operations near the optic chiasm. The BAER is helpful in the diagnosis of acoustic neuroma and brainstem lesions. The SSER tests the integrity of large sensory fibres and their central pathways through dorsal columns, medial lemniscus and thalamus to cortex, and has some specific applications such as monitoring spinal cord function during operations to correct kyphoscoliosis. Note that the slow conduction velocity of pain fibres leads to temporal dispersion of their afferent volley so that they do not contribute to the SSER as usually recorded, which may thus be normal in spite of spinothalamic tract disorder.

Assessment of conduction velocity in central motor pathways

A high voltage, short-duration electrical stimulus or an electromagnetic pulse applied to the scalp over the motor area induces an efferent volley in the pyramidal tract which causes a muscle twitch that can be recorded by EMG. A similar pulse applied to the spinal column stimulates the motor pathway at a segmental level. By subtracting the latency of the muscle twitch evoked from the spinal cord from that induced by stimulation of the motor cortex, the central conduction time and thus conduction velocity can be calculated.

Peripheral nerve conduction velocity

Electrical stimulation of peripheral nerves enables the conduction velocity of their fastest conducting fibres to be measured. The technique is of value in assessing the site of nerve compression, and determining the type and severity of peripheral neuropathy (see Chapter 5). Action potentials of nerve fascicles or single fibres can be recorded by fine intraneural electrodes but this remains a research procedure.

Electromyography (EMG)

Muscle potentials recorded by an intramuscular electrode give characteristic patterns of abnormality in some disorders (Chapter 5). Fibrillations, fasciculation potentials, and positive sharp waves are recorded from denervated muscle while action potentials may be sparser and of larger amplitude because of the sprouting of normal axons to occupy the receptor sites of denervated muscle fibres, thus enlarging the size of surviving motor units (Figs 3.6, 3.7). In myopathies, the muscle potentials are polyphasic and of lower amplitude (Fig. 3.8). The amplitude of the muscle potential evoked by stimulation of motor nerves declines as high frequency stimulation continues in myasthenia gravis, providing an objective record of fatiguability (Fig. 6.4).

In myasthenia, the latency of activation of the single muscle fibres that comprise a motor unit may vary so that muscle potentials recorded by a multipolar electrode during voluntary effort may appear to jump about when displayed on an oscilloscope, a phenomenon known as 'jitter'.

Muscle biopsy

A biopsy may be taken from an affected muscle for histological, histochemical, and electron microscopic examination. It is important that an adequate biopsy of an appropriate muscle be taken by a surgeon experienced in the needs of the pathologist.

Nerve biopsy

A section of peripheral nerve (usually the sural nerve) may be excised to clarify the nature of a peripheral neuropathy. Light and electron microscopic examination may be supplemented by morphometric and teased fibre studies for accurate diagnosis.

General principles of management in hospital

In a hospital setting, the patient's well-being depends on the nursing and paramedical staff at least as much on medical care. Close and courteous collaboration between doctors and nurses, physiotherapists, occupational therapists, speech pathologists, and social workers is essential for the best results. As a general rule, the less time anyone with a degenerative neurological disorder spends in bed the better. Prolonged bedrest will cause a patient with ataxia or Parkinson's disease to become more disabled and will often prolong convalescence. Every person should have the maximum amount of exercise compatible with his or her disability.

Attention to bladder and bowel function, and protection of the skin are obvious essentials. Incontinence of urine or faeces often results from retention with overflow which requires bladder catheterization or disimpaction of faeces, respectively. The doctor should be conversant with the principles of management of respiratory paralysis, coma, and disturbances of fluid balance, electrolytes and nutrition.

Attention should turn to rehabilitation as early as possible. A home visit by a physiotherapist or occupational therapist assists in planning the patient's return, to make life easier by the installation of ramps, railings or other devices to enable disabled persons to function efficiently. All these things seem self-evident but are sometimes neglected. Above all, the aim is to have a happy as well as a healthy person back in the home environment as soon as possible.

The physical comfort of the patient

Simple physical measures may pay dividends. The elevation of a painful or swollen limb, a cradle to keep the weight of bedclothes off a tender or paralysed limb, a foot-drop support or other measures to prevent overstretching of weakened muscles are simple examples. Extension exercises to strengthen the back muscles are important for the relief and prevention of pain in lumbar disc injuries. Traction, mobilization, and some cautious forms of manipulation may be helpful in cervical or lumbar spondylosis. A soft or plastic supportive collar is often used for patients with cervical pain. It is a tautology to say 'cervical collar' since all collars are, by definition, applied to the neck.

Relaxation therapy, with or without biofeedback, is a useful adjuvant to treatment of patients with tension headache and other conditions accompanied by overcontraction of muscles, particularly those of the jaw and face.

Specific therapy

The role of neurosurgery in the management of neurological disorders is beyond the scope of the present text which will concentrate on medical treatments in use.

Medications and procedures shared with other fields of medicine

Analgesics

Antibiotics and antiviral agents (Chapter 19)

Anticoagulants (see Chapter 15)

Vitamins

(1) Thiamine   Thiamine is used for Wernicke's encephalopathy, and some cases of peripheral neuropathy.

(2) Hydroxocobalamin   This forms cyanocobalamin (Vitamin B_{12}) in the body. It is used in tobacco–alcohol amblyopia and Leber's optic atrophy, and for mental changes, subacute combined degeneration or peripheral neuropathy caused by defective absorption of Vitamin B_{12}.

(3) Vitamin E   Some cases of spinocerebellar degeneration are associated with Vitamin E deficiency.

(4) Folate   Folic acid deficiency may be found in patients on long-term anticonvulsant therapy.

Corticosteroids

Indications

(1) Cerebral oedema　Extracellular oedema — postoperative or surrounding tumours — responds to high dosage steroids; for example, dexamethasone, 16–64 mg daily, in divided doses. Intracellular oedema after stroke does not respond to this therapy.

(2) Temporal arteritis (see Chapter 22).

(3) Brachial radiculitis (neuralgic amyotrophy).

(4) Acute herpes zoster　Steroids can be given in addition to acyclovir: 400–800 mg, five times daily, or by half-hour intravenous infusions of 10 mg/kg solution, 8-hourly (Chapter 19).

(5) Polymyositis (Chapter 6).

(6) Tuberculous meningitis　When CSF protein is high corticosteroids are administered in association with antituberculous therapy (Chapter 19).

(7) Myasthenia gravis: resistant cases (Chapter 6).

(8) Acute demyelination　Oral steroids have not proven to be as effective as intramuscular injection of ACTH, 40 U daily for 4 weeks, in the management of an acute relapse of multiple sclerosis. Recently 'pulsed' methylprednisolone, 0.5–1.0 g given by intravenous infusion daily for 5 days, or at third daily intervals in decreasing dosage, has been shown to hasten recovery from a relapse.

(9) Bell's palsy　The value of steroids in the acute phase of Bell's palsy remains controversial. The rationale is to reduce oedema of the facial nerve in the styloid canal.

(10) Relapsing or progressive peripheral neuropathy (see Chapter 5).

(11) Cerebral vasculitis

Immunosuppressant agents

Used in polyarteritis nodosa, systemic lupus erythematosis and other connective tissue diseases, and in some cases of polymyositis, chronic demyelinating peripheral neuropathy, and myasthenia gravis (Chapters 5, 6).

Plasmapheresis (plasma exchange).

(1) Acute phase of Guillain-Barré disease   Plasma exchange is useful when used within 10 days of onset if the disease is progressive and severe (Chapter 5).

(2) Myasthenic crisis (Chapter 6).

(3) Some cases of chronic demyelinating neuropathy (Chapter 5).

Gamma globulin infusion

Used for some resistant cases of myasthenia gravis (Chapter 6).

Medications and procedures used chiefly in neurology

Note that medication should be started with a low dose to minimize the possibility of side-effects.

Pain syndromes

(1) Lightning (stabbing) pains (e.g. trigeminal neuralgia).
(a) Carbamazepine (Tegretol), 100–400 mg three times daily.
(b) Baclofen (Lioresal), 10–20 mg three times daily.

(2) Constant (burning or pressing) pains (e.g. post-herpetic neuralgia, chronic daily headaches). Amitriptyline (Tryptanol, Laroxyl), 10–150 mg *nocte*. Note that the blood levels of amitriptyline may vary ten-fold with the same dose per kg body-weight in different patients so that dosage must be increased slowly and adjusted for the tolerance of the individual.

(3) Intractable pains
(a) Psychological management.
(b) Transcutaneous electrical stimulation (TENS).
(c) Acupuncture.
(d) Analgesics.
(e) Epidural morphine in selected cases.
(f) Surgical procedures in selected cases.

(4) Episodic headache (Chapter 23)

(a) Therapy for acute migraine.

    (i)   Early administration of: metoclopramide (Maxolon), 10 mg intravenously, intramuscularly, or orally; aspirin, 600 mg; ergotamine tartrate, 1–2 mg orally, rectally, or by inhalation.

    (ii) Dihydroergotamine, 1.0 mg intramuscularly, 8-hourly.

    (iii) Naproxen, 250 mg, two tablets three times daily.

(b) Prophylactic (interval) therapy

    (i)   Beta-blockers, e.g. non-selective: propranolol (Inderal), 40–120 mg, twice a day; timolol (Blocadren), 5–10 mg three times daily; or selective beta-1 blockers: atenolol (Tenormin), 50–100 mg daily; metoprolol (Betaloc, Lopresor), 50–100 mg daily.

    (ii) Pizotifen (Sandomigran), 0.5 mg, 2–6 tablets *nocte*.

    (iii) Naproxen, 250 mg, one or two tablets twice daily.

    (iv) Calcium channel-blocking agents (see Chapter 22).

    (v) Methysergide (Deseril), 1–2 mg three times daily.

    (vi) For resistant cases, the MAO inhibitor phenelzine (Nardil) 15 mg two or three times daily, may be used with due precautions.

(5) Cluster headache

(a) Episodic

    (i)   Ergotamine tartrate, 2 mg *nocte* (for nocturnal cluster pain).

    (ii) Methysergide (Deseril), 2 mg three times daily.

    (iii) Prednisone, 60–75 mg daily, with reducing dosage (see Chapter 19).

    (iv) Oxygen inhalation (for acute attack).

(b) Chronic

    (i)   Lithium carbonate, 250 mg two or three times daily with monitoring of blood levels.

    (ii) Calcium channel-blockers.

    (iii) Surgical procedures (rarely).

(c) Chronic paroxysmal hemicrania (CPH)

Indomethacin (Indocid) 25 mg three times daily.

Epilepsy (see Chapter 16)

(1) Partial (focal) and generalized (tonic–clonic, grand mal*) seizures*

(a) Carbamazepine (Tegretol), 100 mg and 200 mg tablets, syrup (100 mg/5 ml). Usual dose adult: 100–400 mg three times daily; children 15–20 mg/kg per day. Dosage to achieve blood levels 20–50 μmol/l, i.e. 3–8 μg/ml.

(b) Phenytoin (Dilantin) 50 mg tablets, 30 mg/5 ml suspension, capsules of 30 mg or 100 mg. Usual dose 100–200 mg twice daily: 6 mg/kg per day for adults and 10 mg/kg per day for children. The required blood levels are 40–80 µmol/l; i.e. 10–20 µg/ml.

(c) Sodium valproate (Epilim) 100 mg, 200 mg (enteric coated tablets), and 500 mg (enteric coated tablets); 200 mg/5 ml liquid or syrup. Usual dose 200–500 mg, three times daily. The blood levels are irrelevant.

(d) Barbiturates

   (i)   Phenobarbitone, 30 mg tablets. Usual dose: 30–90 mg twice daily.
   (ii) Methylphenobarbitone (Prominal), 30, 60, and 200 mg tablets. Usual dose: 60–200 mg twice daily.
   (iii) Primidone (Mysoline), 250 mg tablets. Usual dose: 250–500 mg twice daily. Blood levels are of little help in assessing efficacy.

(e) Benzodiazepines

   (i) Clonazepam (Rivotril), 0.5 and 2 mg tablets, drops: 2.5 mg in 1 ml. Usual dose is 0.5–2.0 mg two or three times daily.
   (ii) Clobazam (Frisium), 10 mg tablets. Usual dose 10 mg two or three times daily as add-on therapy. Blood levels are unnecessary.

(2) Minor generalized seizures (petit mal *absences*)

(a) Sodium valproate, as above.

(b) Clonazepam, as above.

(c) Ethosuximide (Zarontin), 250 mg capsules, syrup, or 250 mg in 5 ml. Blood levels are unnecessary.

(3) Myoclonus

(a) Sodium valproate, as above.

(b) Clonazepam, as above.

(c) Serotonin precursors may be used for post-hypoxic myoclonus or progressive myoclonic epilepsy.

(4) Status epilepticus

(a) Clonazepam, 1 mg in 2 ml bolus or continuous intravenous infusion.

(b) Diazepam, 10 mg in 2 ml bolus or continuous intravenous infusion.

(c) Phenobarbitone sodium, 200 mg in 1 ml, given intramuscularly.

(d) Phenytoin (Dilantin) 100 mg in 2 ml, or 250 mg in 5 ml intravenously, after a loading dose of 15–18 mg/kg infused over 1 h. Phenytoin should never be given intramuscularly.

(e) Thiopentone (Pentothal), intravenously in resistant cases.

Narcolepsy

Special authority is usually required to prescribe these stimulant drugs.
(a) Methylphenidate (Ritalin), 10 mg two or three times daily.
(b) Dexamphetamine (Dexedrine), 5 mg, 1–2 tablets two or three times daily.
(c) Amphetamine (Benzedrine), 5 mg, 1–2 tablets two or three times daily.

Cataplexy

Imipramine (Tofranil), 25 mg three times daily.

Tremor

(1) Essential tremor, action tremor   Alcohol is allowable in socially acceptable amounts and no treatment is required in most cases.
(a) Propranolol, 40–120 mg two or three times daily.
(b) Primidone, 250 mg, 0.5–2 tablets twice daily.
(c) Diazepam, 5 mg, 1–2 tablets three times daily.

(2) Resting tremor of Parkinson's disease
(a) Benzhexol (Artane), tablets of 2 and 5 mg; the usual dose is 1–5 mg three times daily.
(b) Orphenadrine (Disipal), 50 mg tablets; the usual dose is 50 mg three times daily.
(c) Benztropine (Cogentin), 2 mg tablets, dosage 1–2 tablets twice daily.
(d) Stereotactic thalamotomy for unilateral tremor in some cases.

(3) Rubral (red nucleus, 'wing-beating') tremor, intention tremor and hemiballismus
(a) Clonazepam, 0.5–2.0 mg two or three times daily.
(b) Thioridazine (Melleril), 10 mg and 25 mg tablets, dosage 10–50 mg two or three times daily.
(c) Stereotactic thalamotomy in some cases.

Parkinson's disease

(1) Anticholinergic agents   As listed above for tremor. Start with very small doses in the elderly.

(2) Dopamine-releasing agent   Amantadine, 100 mg capsules. Usual dose, 100 mg morning and at midday.

(3) Dopamine precursor   Levodopa + decarboxylase inhibitor in one of two preparations:
(a) Levodopa + carbidopa tablets in the ratios: 100 mg/10 mg, 100 mg/25 mg, and 250 mg/25 mg (Sinemet).
(b) Levodopa + benserazide, 200 mg/50 mg tablets, or capsules in the ratios 50 mg/12.5 mg, 100 mg/25 mg, 200 mg/50 mg (Madopar).

Whichever preparation is used, start with a small dose containing 50–100 mg levodopa and increase the dose slowly to that required to improve performance without inducing involuntary movements or confusion.

(4) Dopamine agonist   Bromocriptine (Parlodel), 2.5 mg tablets, or capsules of 5 mg and 10 mg. It is used as adjuvant therapy with levodopa or as the primary agent in some cases. Start with low doses and increase slowly to avoid side-effects (see Chapter 11).

(5) MAO B inhibitor   Dopamine may be transformed to noradrenaline with the aid of dopamine-hydroxylase or to 3-methoxydopamine by catechol-O-methyl transferase and thence to homovanillic acid by monoamine oxidase B. Deprenyl (Eldepryl) inhibits MAO B, thus prolonging the life and action of dopamine. Since deprenyl has little effect on MAO A, there is no need for the restriction on diet and drugs essential for patients on MAO A inhibitors. At present, deprenyl is available for use only in selected patients by permission of the Commonwealth Department of Health.

Deprenyl comes as 2.5 mg and 10 mg tablets. Added to L-dopa therapy in resistant cases, starting with 2.5 mg daily and slowly increasing to 10 mg daily if necessary.

Intracerebral adrenal implants are now being studied.

Choreoathetosis (including tardive dyskinesia)

(a) Diazepam (Valium), 2, 5, and 10 mg tablets. Usual dose: 2–10 mg three times daily.
(b) Clonazepam (Rivotril), 0.5 and 2 mg tablets. Usual dose: 0.5–2.0 mg twice daily.
(c) Thioridazine (Melleril), 10 and 25 mg tablets. Usual dose: 10–50 mg two or three times daily.

(d) Tetrabenazine (Nitoman), 25 mg tablets. Use is restricted to severe cases, e.g. Huntington's chorea. One tablet two or three times daily.

Dystonia

(a) Benztropine (Cogentin), 2 mg tablets. Usual dose: 2–4 mg twice daily. An injectable form (2 mg in 2 ml) is available for intravenous use in acute dystonia, e.g. that which sometimes follows the use of phenothiazine drugs.

(b) Benzhexol (Artane), 2 and 5 mg tablets; dosage 5–10 mg three times daily. Higher doses have been used in young patients with success.

Gilles de la Tourette syndrome

(a) Clonidine (Catapres), tablets of 100 and 150 μg. Usual dose: one tablet three times daily.

(b) Haloperidol (Serenace, Pacedol, Haldol), tablets of 0.5, 1.5 and 5 mg. Usual dose: 1.5–5 mg three times daily.

(c) Pimozide (Orap), 2 mg tablets. Usual dose: 2 mg two or three times daily.

Spasticity and flexor spasms

(a) Baclofen (Lioresal), 10 and 25 mg tablets. Usual dose: 10–25 mg three times daily.

(b) Diazepam (Valium), 2, 5 and 10 mg tablets. Usual dose: 5–10 mg three times daily.

Multiple sclerosis

(1) Acute relapse   ACTH, 40 U daily for 20–30 days, or pulsed methylprednisolone therapy of 500-1000 mg by intravenous infusion over 30 min every three days, with reducing dosage over a course of six weeks, or as five daily infusions, described earlier in this chapter.

(2) Interval therapy with corticosteroids and immunosuppressive agents has not proved to be of benefit.

(3) Symptomatic treatment
(a) Spasticity — Baclofen or diazepam, as above.
(b) Fatigue — Amantadine (Symmetrel), 100 mg capsules. Dosage: one

capsule two or three times daily has been recommended but is of doubtful benefit.

(c) Urgency of micturition — Penthienate bromide (Monodral), 5 mg tablets. Usual dose: 5 mg three times daily.

(d) Tremor — Clonazepam and other agents as listed under tremor.

Cerebral vascular disease

(1) Transient ischaemic attacks　Aspirin, 50, 100, or 300 mg tablets. Enteric-coated tablets containing 650 mg. The dose of 650 mg twice daily is of proven efficacy in normotensive males. The efficacy of lower doses is currently under trial.

(2) Cerebral embolism of cardiac origin　Anticoagulant agents, heparin initially and warfarin for a period of up to six months, are used in conventional doses.

(3) Completed stroke　The infusion of 500 ml of 10% glycerol in normal saline, administered over 4 h daily for 6 consecutive days, has been reported to reduce mortality in the first week.

Vertigo

Note that these agents may cause acute dystonic reactions requiring intravenous injection of 2 mg benztropine. Long-term use may cause tardive dyskinesia.

(a) Prochlorperazine (Stemetil), 5 mg tablets or suppositories of 5 mg and 25 mg. Injections or suppositories given as required for acute vertigo. Usual oral dose: 5 mg three times daily.

(b) Thiethylperazine (Torecan), 6.5 mg base tablets or suppositories. Injection 6.5 mg base in 1 ml. Injections or suppositories are given as required for acute vertigo. Usual oral dose: 6.5 mg base three times daily.

(c) Diuretics, potassium supplements and vasodilator agents are used for interval therapy of Menière's disease but are of doubtful value.

Myasthenia gravis

(1) Anticholinesterase agents

(a) Edrophonium (Tensilon). Injection of 10 mg in 1 ml, diluted to 10 ml in normal saline and injected intravenously, slowly over 2 min, as a diagnostic test.

(b) Prostigmine, 15 mg tablets or injections of 1 mg. Usual oral dose: 1-2 tablets, 3-hourly.

(c) Pyridostigmine (Mestinon), tablets of 10, 60, and 180 mg (sustained release). Usual dose: 60 mg, 1-2 tablets, every 4-8 h.

(2) Potassium-retaining agents These are out of fashion at the moment but can be very useful in resistant cases.

Potassium supplements (e.g. K-lyte, Span K), 1-2 tablets three times daily. Triamterene (Dytac), 100 mg tablets, once or twice daily. Spironolactone (Aldactone A), 25 mg tablets, 1-4 tablets three times daily. (Note: serum electrolytes should be checked as these agents can cause hyperkalaemia.)

(3) Ephedrine 30-60 mg three times daily can be used as adjuvant therapy.

(4) Plasmapheresis or gamma globulin infusions may be indicated in severe cases. Corticosteroids are prescribed in some cases after thymectomy or in some patients resistant to other forms of therapy. Guanidine (5-10 mg/kg, three times daily) is used for Eaton-Lambert syndrome (myasthenia associated with malignant disease). Immunosuppressants have been advocated for severe cases.

Myotonia

(a) Quinine sulphate, 300 mg tablets. Usual dose: one tablet once or twice daily.

(b) Phenytoin (Dilantin), capsules of 100 mg. Usual dose: 100 mg three times daily.

(c) Procainamide (Pronestyl) is used for some severe cases but can produce a lupus-like syndrome.

Pseudomyotonia, muscle cramps

(a) Carbamazepine (Tegretol), 100 and 200 mg tablets. Usual dose: 100-200 mg three times daily.

(b) Quinine sulphate, as above.

Reference

Johnson R.T. (1986) *Current Therapy in Neurologic Disease 1985-86*. B.C. Decker, Ontario.

Index